"Richard Rosen is one of the most thoughtful, generous, funny, humble, and researched fellas that I know. *Yoga FAQ* is a testimony to Richard's character as a man and diligence as a yogi. The content is for anyone that is not satisfied with being a blind follower. Richard has done the research and held the debates to debunk unsubstantiated yoga myths that we deem as fact. His curiosity and inability to be satisfied with superficiality have brought us a text that will leave many of us scratching our heads and maybe even feeling a little defensive as our beliefs are being tested. This is important stuff for anyone that craves to see what is below the surface of the yogic teachings. If we keep asking the questions, maybe we might get a glimpse of how these practices can bring about true happiness."

—COLLEEN SAIDMAN, author of *Yoga for Life*

"Richard Rosen has crafted a delightful book that showcases equally both his academic knowledge about yoga and his gentle sense of humor. *Yoga FAQ* is a clear resource that helps us to formulate and understand our big questions about yoga and spiritual practice. I felt as if I were tucking into the personal story of Mr. Rosen's own journey studying yoga — and the trip was intriguing and fun. Highly recommended for all levels of students and especially for yoga teachers."

—JUDITH HANSON LASATER, PhD, PT, author of *Relax and Renew* and *Yoga Body*

"*Yoga FAQ* is an indispensable addition to any yoga enthusiast's shelf. Fact-filled and scholarly, this book makes you feel like the author is sitting across from you, sipping tea and patiently answering your every query. Richard Rosen has a remarkable way of honoring the great traditions and the newer expressions of yoga, with just enough humor and irreverence to keep you turning page after page."

—ANNIE CARPENTER, creator of SmartFLOW Yoga

"Richard Rosen is one of the wisest, warmest, and funniest writers I know, as well as being one of the most skilled and learned yoga teachers in America. In this book he brings all of those qualities to bear on some of the topics that routinely confuse students of yoga, new and old. A great service."

—MARK SINGLETON, author of *Yoga Body: The Origins of Modern Posture Practice* and *Roots of Yoga*

YOGA FAQ

YOGA FAQ

Almost Everything
You Need to Know
About Yoga—from
Asanas to Yamas

RICHARD ROSEN

SHAMBHALA
Boulder
2017

Shambhala Publications, Inc.
4720 Walnut Street
Boulder, Colorado 80301
www.shambhala.com

© 2017 by Richard Rosen

9 8 7 6 5 4 3 2 1

FIRST EDITION
Printed in the United States of America

∞ This edition is printed on acid-free paper that meets the
American National Standards Institute z39.48 Standard.
♻ This book is printed on 30% postconsumer recycled paper.
For more information please visit www.shambhala.com.

Distributed in the United States by Penguin Random House LLC
and in Canada by Random House of Canada Ltd

Designed by Steve Dyer

LIBRARY OF CONGRESS CATALOGING-IN-PUBLICATION DATA
Names: Rosen, Richard, author.
Title: Yoga FAQ: almost everything you need to know
about yoga—from Asanas to Yamas / Richard Rosen.
Description: First Edition. | Boulder: Shambhala, 2017. |
Includes bibliographical references and index.
Identifiers: LCCN 2016011783 | ISBN 9781611801736 (pbk.: alk. paper)
Subjects: LCSH: Hatha yoga.
Classification: LCC BL1238.56.H38 R673 2016 | DDC613.7/046—dc23
LC record available at https://lccn.loc.gov/2016011783

Many of the old Hatha Yoga books open with a salutation delivered by the book's author or compiler. The purpose is to acknowledge his indebtedness to his teacher, whether he be human or divine, who's credited as the ultimate source of the material about to be presented. The salutation might begin with the Sanskrit word *shri*, which has a wealth of meaning—"radiance, splendor, glory, beauty, grace, prosperity, success, auspiciousness," among many others—though typically it's meant as a title of respect, even reverence, for the man or deity so invoked.

In keeping with this long tradition, *shri*, I'd like to dedicate this book to the memory of Georg Feuerstein (1947–2012). Georg was never officially my "guru"; I seriously doubt he would have accepted that role. But over the fifteen years I knew him, that's how I secretly thought of him, and still do today. Hardly a day goes by that I don't look into one of his many books to draw inspiration from the immense store of his wisdom. He'll be quoted and referenced often with great affection and respect in the pages that follow.

O Parvati, nothing is so fruitful, pleasing, subtle, mysterious, enlightening, and lovely as yoga.

"Seed of Yoga" (*Yoga Bija*), verse 81

Contents

Foreword

FRIENDSHIP IS ONE OF THE great human gifts, and a long, enduring friendship is sheer beauty and grace. Richard Rosen has been my dear friend for more than thirty years, and all that time I have depended on him for advice, wisdom, understanding, and just plain fun.

So what is he offering up in this latest book? One afternoon a few years ago, we sat in his book-lined office and talked about all the misconceptions circulating in the yoga community. I suggested to him that his next book should address these modern-day misconceptions, and now, after hours and hours of research, long days huddled over his computer, and — as he tells me — three missed deadlines, he's finally delivered what I asked for.

The book starts by addressing some of the most basic yoga questions, and Richard's research leads to some startling discoveries. What is yoga? Where did it start? How did it get to the West? What is the relationship of how and why it is practiced today to how and why it was practiced at different times throughout history? Is it a beneficial practice for the modern world, and what can we expect to get from yoga?

Some elementary school kids in the United States learn yoga in school, and if you ask them what it is, they usually come up with answers like, it's something that makes you calm, relaxed, and flexible. They will imitate some postures and sitting meditation. Where did they get this impression? If you ask an average yoga teacher what yoga is, you usually get a little talk on "union" and how the practice is five thousand years old. They may have some poses and sequences of poses that they practice and teach, along with some information on breathing and meditation. Where did they get this information and these practices, and what relationship do they have with the great river of yoga knowledge and techniques?

Without much more than an ounce of questioning we have acquired so much misinformation on yoga from our teachers. It is easy to hand down these myths and stories that twist and turn from their original form and meaning, and often lead us away from the essence of a specific lesson or practice. This may not lessen the validity of what we have been practicing or teaching as a whole, but it often clouds the wisdom we could be gathering from the masters of the past. Where would the world of yoga be if we did not stand on the shoulders of yoga giants?

If the first real concrete mention of yoga, as Richard notes in his book, is in the *Katha Upanishad*, some 2,500 years ago, it becomes an immediate necessity to ask, what was this yoga being used for and what were the techniques employed? Also, one wants to find out about the culture and time it is set in to comprehend its relative meaning. Are any of these practices followed today, and if so do they have any relevancy for us? How about the *Yoga Sutra*? What is this compilation of pithy statements about, and how does it apply to our modern yoga practice and our modern life?

Richard digs deep into the history and art of yoga to set us straight on many of the mistaken myths that we pass among ourselves. He also answers some profound questions that shed light on where the world of yoga might want to travel and explore. There are some forgotten practices, or possibly purposely left-out practices, that may not have been suitable for the Western mind and body, or for the masses. As we become more adept in yoga, these lost techniques might reveal themselves to be indispensable. As our perspectives shift, from our hopefully ever-evolving studies and questions, we need specific tools to aid our exploration.

Albert Einstein was once asked what he would do if given an hour to solve a problem — how would he go about it? His reply was that he would spend fifty-five minutes figuring out what the most essential question was, and then spend the last five minutes answering the question. What are the yoga questions and what tools do we need to answer them? Richard makes it abundantly clear that at various times in the history of yoga, the questions and desired outcomes have changed, and the methods and techniques to solve them have also shifted. For instance, what was the general purpose, philosophy, and methodology of the *Hatha Yoga Pradipika*, and how did it differ from the *Yoga Sutra*? Some five hundred years later, the *Pradipika* might be talking about a different subject with different goals in mind.

In my tool cabinet, I have many different manuals for the different machines in our house, and it would be foolish for me to read my dishwasher's manual for my car stereo problems. Richard unearths these original yoga texts and unravels their historical context and meaning so that we can use this information for our own pursuits. What are your questions and goals, and what manuals can help shed light on solving your problems and reaching your goals?

Even though there is something for everyone in yoga, the specific style you study and the methodologies it utilizes can be very different from other schools. Where did all of these different schools of yoga come from, and what specifically are they good for? As we go beyond the superficial layers of our modern-day practice, we see the infinite beauty of this art and the variety of approaches and systems that rally around the questions of "who am I?" "how can I be happy?" and "how can I dwell in a state of inner peace?" Some modern schools divorce themselves from anything "spiritual" and focus instead on a yoga butt. It is not that these schools are right or wrong; it is just questionable whether or not they have anything to do with yoga.

When our eyes are opened, it gives us so much more joy, clarity, and renewed curiosity on the yoga path. The mystery of our mind, body, and soul and the possibility of Self-realization are always intriguing, and it's a gift to find any text, sequence, or technique that can illuminate another door to yet another room of beauty and joy on this path. In this book, Richard has done a lot of the heavy lifting for us. He shows us where many of us have made false assumptions about yoga and how these assumptions can impede our path to liberation.

As we rid ourselves of this misinformation, we are able to fully receive the wisdom of the past. Now, we have no excuse but to clean up our act and read this authoritative book — and relieve some of our ignorance. Once again, I thank you, Richard, for your curiosity, your love, your intelligence, your diligence, but most of all for your friendship.

— RODNEY YEE

Preface

THIS IS A BOOK OF QUESTIONS about yoga and my proposed answers to them. I want to emphasize right out of the gate that the answers I give are *my* answers, not *the* answers. When, as is very often the case, the answer is a matter of debate, usually between Western scholars and Indian traditionalists and their Western supporters—How old is yoga? Where does Sanskrit come from? Who was Patanjali?—I've tried to represent all the arguments fairly. Sometimes I do a good job, but other times I can't help myself, and my Western bias shows through: yoga is NOT five thousand years old; Sanskrit is derived from proto-Indo-European and Vedic sources, NOT heaven and the gods; and NOTHING is known about Patanjali. (We'll come back to all this later in the book.) I apologize in advance to anyone I rub the wrong way.

I have caveats (Latin *cavere*, "to be on guard") about the book's title and its subtitle. The title suggests that the questions addressed herein are all "frequently asked," and this is true for most but not all of them. Consider, for example, the very first question in the book: Is yoga appropriate for Westerners? Some very smart people think it isn't, including Swiss psychiatrist Carl Jung (1875–1961) and Polish cultural philosopher Jean Gebser (1905–1973). It's not likely you'll *ever* hear this question asked in a yoga class, on the off chance that Carl and Jean turn out to be right. Let's just say that if any of the questions in this book are not frequently asked, in my opinion they should be.

Then there's the subtitle, which promises that "almost everything" you need to know about yoga will be found within these pages. Be advised, though, that the word "almost" is used purposefully. Since yoga has been around for at least two-and-a-half millennia (but NOT five millennia), the subject matter that has accumulated about it is, not surprisingly, quite extensive, not to mention bewilderingly contradictory. To deliver even "almost" everything would require many more pages than I've been allotted; for example, Dr. Feuerstein's invaluable survey of the subject, *The Yoga Tradition,* checks in at more than seven hundred pages and doesn't even cover "modern" yoga (a subject he wasn't much interested in). This book answers "almost everything" you need to know about yoga within the bounds of the questions I've posed.

You may find yourself disagreeing with one of my answers here and there, or you may come to my daughter's conclusion about most everything I say—that I simply don't know what I'm talking about. I'm fine with that, but I hope you'll use any disagreement as the starting point for an investigation of your own. To help you along I've provided reading lists at the end of this book. The volumes that I recommend are all in my possession, and I've either read them or told myself I will read them someday (to justify my crammed bookshelves).

You may have a couple questions of your own. For instance, where did I get the questions I ask? Though I've cautioned that a few may not exactly be "frequently asked," most of them are quite common. In general, the basic questions (e.g., what is a *sutra*?) are the ones I've posed myself, during my thirty-six years as a yoga student and teacher. The more involved questions derive from a poll I conducted among the world's greatest students: mine.

You might also wonder how I chose what to include and what to leave out. The first and fifth chapters, on yoga in general and Hatha Yoga in particular, were no-brainers. The third and fourth chapters, on the Veda, the Upanishads, and the *Yoga Sutra,* were not quite slam-dunks, but given the importance of these texts to the origin and development of yoga, I could hardly leave them out.

The second chapter, on Sanskrit, was the toughest call. The "language of yoga," as my friend Nicolai Bachman has dubbed it, is not only widely misunderstood but also routinely mispronounced. I truly believe that if we're going to use Sanskrit at all, we should at least try to use it properly, out of respect for one of the oldest languages still in everyday use. When I set out to write this book, I decided I would try to bring some clarity to the situation, as much as I could with my kindergarten-level Sanskrit ("see Patanjali run"), but I wasn't sure that anyone besides myself and a few Sanskrit nerds would be interested. So I drafted the chapter and gave it to a few of my students (I knew they wouldn't pull any punches). The consensus was unanimous: include the chapter. So I did.

Since I couldn't cover everything, I'm sure that you'll find yourself exclaiming, perhaps more than once, "How in the world could he leave *that* out?" For example, while I'm very interested in Hatha Yoga (which not coincidentally is the longest chapter in the book), I'm not especially interested in Karma Yoga and Bhakti Yoga, the practices of unselfish service and unstinting devotion, so you won't find any questions concerning them in this book.

I suppose the most egregious omission are the questions I haven't posed about the "Lord's Song," the *Bhagavad Gita*, considered by many people to be one of the classics of world spiritual literature, and surely as well-known among Western students as the *Yoga Sutra*. (Please refer to page 85 for a note regarding *Yoga Sutra* [singular] vs. *Sutras* [plural].) It's not that I lacked material; there are at least a baker's dozen *Gita* translations and commentaries in my library. I pondered long and hard about this one, but in the end I had to admit to myself that, despite its glowing reputation, the poem just doesn't interest me very much. So you'll find hardly a mention here of the warrior Arjuna and his charioteer Krishna, the former's pre-battle identity crisis or the latter's win-one-for-the-Gipper pep talk.

After eighteen months of research on this book, and almost four decades of personal inquiry, I can safely say with some authority that there are an awful lot of questions about yoga. Many of these questions have answers, often more than one. Many more questions haven't the inkling of an answer, either because we don't have enough historical information to answer them yet or because they are fundamentally unanswerable. But all of these questions, whatever their concern, boil down to one ultimate question, which is, "Who am I?"

The "who" here of course isn't the "who" on your driver's license—

the "who" with the unflattering photo and the low-balled weight. No, this "who" is someone else we all know in our heart-of-hearts but somehow in our heads have mostly forgotten, much to our detriment—not to mention that of our little planet. I'm not going to say more about this question right now; we'll return to it in the following pages. But you might want to keep the following words from the Indian sage Ramana Maharshi (1879–1950) in the back of your heart as you read along.

> Every living being longs always to be happy . . . and everyone has the greatest love for himself, which is solely due to the fact that happiness is his real nature. Hence, in order to realize that inherent and untainted happiness . . . it is essential that he should know himself. For obtaining such knowledge the enquiry "Who am I?" in quest for the Self is the best means.
>
> From the essay "Who Am I?" in Arthur Osborne, ed.,
> *The Collected Works of Ramana Maharshi*, p. 39

RICHARD ROSEN
Berkeley, California
January 2016

Acknowledgments

I FIRST WANT TO THANK my editor, Beth Frankl, who could have taught Job a thing or two about patience. For a variety of reasons this book took an inordinate length of time to write; I lost count of missed deadlines. I'll be forever grateful to Beth for generously giving me the time and space to finish this project, with nary a grumpy word spoken.

I'd also like to thank my long-time students, who suggested many of the questions in this book. I'm convinced they are the best students ever.

And, as always, I'd like to acknowledge my teachers (some of whom may not be too pleased with some of the essays following). Everything of value here comes from them; the mistakes are mine alone.

Abbreviations

Sanskrit title (English translation)
Author (AU)/Compiler (C)/Attributed to (AT) · Estimated Date

BU   *Brihad Aranyaka Upanishad* (Great Forest Upanishad)
Anon · ninth century B.C.E.

BYY *Brihad Yogi Yajnavalkya Smṛti* (Great Codex of Yogi Yajnavalkya)
Yajnavalkya (AT) · fourteenth to fifteenth centuries C.E.

CU   *Chandogya Upanishad* (Chanter's Upanishad)
Anon · ninth to seventh centuries B.C.E.

GS   *Gheranda Samhita* (Gheranda's Collection)
Anon · late seventeenth century C.E.

GoS *Goraksha Shataka* (Goraksha's Hundred [Verses])
Goraksha (AT) · twelfth to thirteenth centuries C.E.

HRA *Hatha Ratna Avali* (String of Jewels on Hatha [Yoga])
Shrinivasa Bhatta (AU) · late sixteenth century C.E.

HYP *Hatha Yoga Pradipika* (Light on Forceful Yoga)
Svatmarama (C) · mid-fifteenth century C.E.

JP   *Joga Pradipyaka* (Hindi dialect) (Light on Yoga)
Jayatarama (AU) · 1718 C.E.

KU   *Katha Upanishad*
Anon · fifth century B.C.E.

KJN *Kaula Jnana Nirnaya* (Ascertainment of Kaula Knowledge)
Matsyendra (AT) · mid-eleventh century C.E.

LoY   *Light on Yoga*
       B. K. S. Iyengar (AU) · 1966
       All numbers in parentheses refer to photo plate numbers unless
       otherwise noted.

MU   *Maitri Upanishad* (Friendship Upanishad)
       Anon · third to second century B.C.E.

RJ   *Raja Yoga* / Royal Yoga (cf. *Yoga Sutra*)
       Vivekananda (AU) · 1896

RV   *Rig Veda* (Knowledge of Praise)
       Anon · dates much debated, see Chapter 3

SS   *Shiva Samhita* (Shiva's Collection)
       Anon · seventeenth century

SSP   *Siddha Siddhanta Paddhati* (Doctrine of the Adepts' Tracks)
       Goraksha (AT) · eleventh to twelfth centuries C.E.

VS   *Vasishtha Samhita* (Vasishtha's Collection)
       Vasishtha (AT) · fourteenth to fifteenth centuries C.E.

YS   *Yoga Sutra* (Yoga Threads)
       Patanjali (C) · fifth century B.C.E to third century C.E.

YY   *Yoga Yajnavalkya* (Yajnavalkya's Yoga)
       Yajnavalkya (AT) · twelfth century C.E.

In what follows, I refer to Classical Yoga (Patanjali's *Yoga Sutra*, also known
as Raja Yoga, Patanjali Yoga) as CY.

YOGA FAQ

1

UNION
What Is Yoga?

Now, the teachings of yoga
(*atha yoga anushasanam*)

Yoga Sutra I.I, translation
by Chip Hartranft

So READS THE VERY FIRST "thread" (*sutra*) of Patanjali's 1,800-year-old yoga outline, the *Yoga Sutra*. It's possibly one of the most famous opening lines in all of Hindu spiritual literature, right up there with, "In the field of righteousness, the field of the Kurus," which sets the scene for the universally revered *Bhagavad Gita*. But still, most beginning students, intent on getting to the good parts of Patanjali's teaching, understandably skip right past the little word "now" (Sanskrit *atha*, pronounced AH-TAH) without a second thought. But wait now! An essential characteristic of the sutra literary style is brevity—out, darned adjective; begone, you adverb—so it's highly likely that *atha* is there for a good reason.

What's so special about "now"? Rutgers professor of Indian religion Edwin Bryant remarks that this "now" indicates to a student picking up the *Yoga Sutra* for the first time that, after searching far and wide in "other philosophical or religious systems," he or she has finally happened upon the way to the Truth-with-a-capital-T.[1] This "now" is, I suppose we could say, a congratulations and a welcome home. It's also an attention-getter: the book's compiler, Patanjali, is announcing, "I'm ready to teach, so listen up."

Nowadays we can flip through the *Yoga Sutra* whenever we please and then put it back on the shelf, but once upon a time embarking on the study of Classical Yoga was serious business. It required a sincere commitment and long period of preparation just to gain access to the actual text and its teaching. At a point determined by the teacher—*atha*, "now"— the novice was deemed qualified for instruction. It must have been an exhilarating moment, when the student left behind her mundane existence and identity and entered her brand-new life as spiritual aspirant. So in this respect, "now" serves as a sign of recognition and acknowledgment.

My Sanskrit-English dictionary describes *atha* as an "auspicious particle," a sort of good-luck blessing. It's uttered at the start of any great undertaking to ensure a successful outcome, whether by a yoga teacher at the beginning of a course of study, or (as one Hindu legend holds) by the Creative Principle, called *Brahma*, at the creation of the universe— though I suppose we'll have to wait and see if it works for our troubled planet. Swami Veda Bharati echoes this blessing aspect of *atha* when he writes: "May the study undertaken, the guidance given and received, and the disciplines observed come to bear their desired results without impediments."[2]

SWAMI/SVAMI

We'll run across several swamis in this book. As you likely already know, a "swami" is a title for a spiritual teacher or scholarly Brahmin. In Chapter 2, we'll learn about something called anglicization, the tendency we English speakers have to make supposedly strange foreign words more comfortable to our eyes and ears. Also in Chapter 2, we'll learn how the pronunciation of the Sanskrit *v* is modified to sound more like a *w* when it follows a consonant in a word.

So, when English speakers hear a Sanskrit speaker say the word spelled s-v-a-m-i, what they hear sounds like "swami." It was only natural then for *svami* to end up in English spoken and spelled as *swami*.

Finally, *atha* whispers a subtle message and reminder for each of us: that all yoga teaching emerges from and ultimately leads us back to the timeless, ever-present NOW. Here, in the timeless present, writes

Patanjali, the "layers and imperfections concealing truth" are "washed away" (YS 4.31), and our authentic Self, "grounded in its very nature" (YS 4.34), is revealed.

Now, I didn't mention that there's one catch. When *atha* appears at the beginning of a sacred text, it is said to be most auspicious if it's spoken aloud. Are you ready now? Repeat after me: *atha, atha, atha.*

YOGI/YOGINI

Let's get some terminology straight before we dive any deeper. Technically, a male practitioner of yoga is a *yogi* (pronounced YOH-gee, the *g* sounds like the *g* in "get"; the second syllable rhymes with "we"), and a female practitioner is a *yogini* (YOH-gee-nee, with the emphasis on the *first* syllable). However, it's acceptable to refer to a male or female practitioner as a yogi, which is the name we'll use in this book.

» *Is yoga appropriate for Westerners?*

> These paths [i.e., of yoga] are inappropriate for Europeans . . . or even detrimental within the European milieu, if for no other reason than because the complete suppression or exclusion of volition is possible only for the few. The contemporary European can scarcely distinguish any longer between effort of will, intensive concentration, and true meditation, since he attempts to direct all of them with his rationality—an attempt that necessarily leads to unfortunate results.
>
> JEAN GEBSER, *The Ever-Present Origin* (1949), p. 243, note 83

Is the practice of yoga inappropriate for Westerners? This is an odd question you won't hear asked much, if at all, in the American yoga community. Why is that? It might be that it just hasn't occurred to anyone. Or the answer might seem obvious: *of course* yoga is appropriate—why else would thirty-six million of us be spending *billions* of dollars every year on yoga classes, books, magazines, and videos, retreats and conferences, yoga gear and clothing, and assorted Hindu geegaws? No doubt these are impressive numbers, but they don't settle the issue, since it's possible that a whole passel of Americans are blissfully but unknowingly engaged in inappropriate behavior—not an uncommon phenomenon.

But why would this question come up in the first place? How could your weekly asana class be considered "inappropriate," even "detrimental"? It seems that some thoughtful people over the past half-century or so, though not yoga teachers themselves, have had serious doubts that Eastern spiritual practices like yoga can be successfully transplanted in the West. Who are these people and what are their objections?

Probably the most famous yoga opponent was Carl Jung (1875–1961), the Swiss psychiatrist, argonaut of the collective unconscious, and founder of the school of analytical psychology. Jung apparently first became interested in Indian philosophy as a teenager after reading the nineteenth-century German philosopher Arthur Schopenhauer, who was heavily influenced by the teachings of the Upanishads—he reportedly named all of his beloved poodles "Atman," the Upanishadic word for the Self. Of the Upanishads, he once wrote:

> From every sentence deep, original, and sublime thoughts arise, and the whole is pervaded by a high and holy and earnest spirit. . . . In the whole world there is no study, except that of the originals, so beneficial and so elevating as that of the *Oupnekhat* [the Latin translation of the Upanishads]. It has been the solace of my life, it will be the solace of my death.[3]

Though he objected to Westerners doing yoga, Jung didn't exactly practice what he preached. He admitted that, during a troubled period of self-analysis, he himself turned to yoga exercises to hold his "emotions in check." But he was careful to add that his purpose was much different from that of the yogi. He would do the exercises only until he had calmed himself enough to resume digging into his unconscious. As soon as he was calm, he abandoned the "restraint" on his emotions and "allowed the images and inner voices to speak afresh." In contrast, said Jung, the yogi does yoga exercises to "obliterate completely the multitude of psychic content and images."[4]

While Jung objected to the practice of yoga, he held Eastern wisdom in high regard, and much of his work, like Schopenhauer's, was influenced by India. In 1938, when the British government invited him to visit there, he readily accepted the opportunity to have an up-close-and-personal look at the source of this wisdom. India was a revelation for Jung. Though he was sixty-three years old and widely traveled, it was his first encounter with what he considered a truly "alien" culture. He commented that India was like a "dream," though reality intruded when he contracted dysentery and spent ten miserable days in a hospital.

What were Jung's objections to Westerners practicing yoga, and more to the point, how much validity, if any, do they have? He based his stance on the premise that Easterners and Westerners experience the world, and themselves, in diametrically opposite ways. Indians are innately introverts, he argued. Their attention is forever turned toward the "inner subjective," the unconscious, and resolutely away from the "outer objective," Nature, which for them has little or no lasting value. The typical Westerner, in Jung's view, is an extrovert; his conscious mind is so strong that it essentially severs, and so alienates him from, his unconscious psychic roots. Westerners direct their attention "outside," away from the subjective and toward Nature, which we then seek to dominate and exploit to our advantage.

So what happens then when a Western extrovert comes face-to-face with introverted Indian yoga? Jung pointed out two general tendencies. Some of us, because we're so completely unconscious of our unconscious, project onto the "alien" East all of our hidden fears and hatreds, and react as we instinctively do whenever we feel threatened.

The rest of us, precisely *because* we're so alienated from our inner lives, which seem empty of anything spiritually good or useful, uncritically assume that saving knowledge can only be found "outside." Rejecting Western spiritual traditions (a rejection that Jung interpreted as a kind of self-avoidance), we fall heels over head in love with yoga, with its tantalizing promise of reintegrating our fragmented psychic pieces and bringing us to "union" with our true Self. The only way we can truly understand and apply yoga's introverted methods, Jung suggested, is if we sit "on a gazelle skin under a Bo-tree" for the rest of our lives, and forget about the stock market, real estate, politics, and our favorite football team—a near impossible task for us hopeless extroverts of the West. Otherwise "yoga in Mayfair or Fifth Avenue, or in any other place which is on the telephone, is a spiritual fake."[5]

Even if Western yoga is fake—and that has yet to be decided—how is it harmful, other than that we may be fooling ourselves (and making fools of ourselves)? Jung quotes a Chinese saying: "If the wrong man uses the right means, the right means will work in the wrong way." He implies that, ironically, when extroverts "do" yoga, yoga will have precisely the opposite of the intended effect: instead of regaining the lost or abandoned portions of our psyches, we'll only strengthen our already crushing Western willfulness and divorce ourselves even further from the unconscious, causing an "absence of instinct, nervousness, disorientation and entanglement in impossible situations and problems."[6] We certainly can't dismiss any of Carl's comments about Westerners and yoga, no matter how much they may sting. I'm pretty sure if pressed, many of our teachers would admit to seeing examples of Western inappropriateness in their students (and themselves, maybe).

But still, I'm also pretty sure that, as we take Indian yoga and carefully and respectfully adapt it to our needs, the question of whether or not we're "right" for yoga will ultimately be answered with a resounding "Yes!"

For the last word on this subject, I'll turn, as I did so many times when he was alive, to Dr. Feuerstein, to see what he has to say about all this. Always an optimist, he assures us that our difficulties with yoga aren't necessarily due to some "psychological incompatibility"; rather, our difficulty is more likely the result of a lack of "self-discipline and understanding," two qualities Dr. Feuerstein possessed in abundance.[7]

» I've always been told, "Yoga means union." What exactly does that mean?

Yoga means union. The union of the individual soul with the Universal Spirit is yoga.

B. K. S. IYENGAR, *The Tree of Yoga* (1988), p. 3

If we were to ask a typical student to render the Sanskrit "yoga" into English, how would she respond? She might decide to go with "yoke" or "join," two words that are cognate with "yoga" through an ancient root (*yuj*). But after more than three decades of wandering about in Yoga Land, I can predict with some confidence that the word she'd come up with, as would most yoga students and teachers, is "union." Much like the popular answer to the question, "How old is yoga?" which for mysterious reasons is almost always given as five thousand years (a claim we'll address shortly), "yoga means union" seems to have been indelibly, even unquestioningly, implanted in our brains. But even though this definition is widely accepted, there are three misconceptions associated with it that are generally overlooked, and in need of correcting.

Yoga as Union-Method

Our first step will be to consult one of the monuments of Western Sanskrit scholarship, *A Sanskrit-English Dictionary,* compiled by the British Orientalist and Sanskritist Monier Monier-Williams (1819–1899). First published in 1872, my reprint of the second, 1899 edition has 186,000 entries spread over more than 1,300 pages and weighing in at eight pounds. In a pinch it could substitute for your average sandbag.

The 360-word "yoga" entry reads like a grab bag of meanings. Some we expect, like "yoke" and "join," found right in the opening line, and our favored "union," listed about a third of the way down. But others we don't. Did you know that "yoga" also means "a remedy, a cure"? That sort of makes sense, but "a trick, fraud" and "deceit" don't seem very yoga-like at all. Neither does "acquisition, gain, profit, wealth," or "a violator of confidence" and "spy."

Be that as it may, what interests us most here is that "yoga" is also defined as a "means, way, manner, method." This usage likely refers back to the time, at least 2,500 years ago (and no doubt even earlier), when horse-drawn chariots were used both on ceremonial occasions and in military operations. These war wagons typically carried two passengers (though there were larger ones that could accommodate up to seven), a charioteer and a warrior, the latter usually wielding a bow and arrow, though sometimes a long spear. The horses that supplied the motive power in battle weren't your docile plow pullers from down on the farm; rather, they were feisty, often uncooperative, and always unpredictable beasts.

It was the charioteer's job to yoke these equines to the chariot, and no doubt this required a good deal of skill and a time-tested method to ensure success; after all, it wouldn't do, in the heat of battle, to have the horses break loose and go galloping off, leaving the chariot and its now sitting-duck occupants behind. So we can say that originally yoga had two equally important, related meanings: the one everybody knows indicates its goal, that is, joining or union; the second acknowledges that this could be achieved only by applying the proper method.

Now we can draw an analogy between our practice and the charioteer's job. We both have a goal we hope to achieve, which is "union" (however that's defined). But by itself it's only half the story. The single word "union" fails to recognize one of the central tenets of the traditional teaching; that is to say, as with any goal we have in our sights, whether it's harnessing a team of rowdy horses or doing the same, figuratively speaking, to the unruly "fluctuations" (*vrtti*) of our minds (see Chapter 4), we must of necessity have a practical means to reach it.

The Sanskrit-English dictionary supplies us with several suitable words that may be appended to "union" to complete the English equivalent of the Sanskrit "yoga." We have "application," "performance," "means," "expedient," "way," and "method." I'll let you pick one for yourself, but I prefer "union-method," which is how this book will define "yoga" in most contexts from here on out.

THE "IMAGE OF THE CHARIOT" (*RATHA KALPANA*)

One of the best known Upanishadic parables is called the *ratha kalpana*, the "image of the chariot." It's found in the *Katha Upanishad* (see 3.3–11), which is the earliest surviving text that contains a concrete reference to yoga practice. The parable is set within a fantastic frame story relating the adventure of a precocious youngster, Naciketas (meaning, "I don't know"), who's consigned to the underworld by his father in a moment of pique. Once there, because of a serious breach in hospitality, he's given three boons by the realm's presiding deity, Yama, the "Restrainer." The boy's first two wishes, to be returned to the upper world and his father's good graces and to have revealed to him the meaning of the "heavenly" sacrificial fire (1.13), are readily granted by Yama.

But the deity's willingness to accommodate Naciketas comes to an abrupt halt with wish number three. The boy wants to know—and who better to ask than Yama?—what happens to a person after death. "Oh," replies the deity, "that's a tough one, not even the other gods are sure about the answer." He begs the boy to pick something else, and offers him one worldly temptation after another: livestock, elephants, gold, estates, long life, and, at last, after all this was turned down, anything his little heart desires. Naciketas, though, refuses to be swayed by what he disparagingly calls "ephemeral things" (1.26), and insists on learning about the afterlife.

Why does Yama try to derail Naciketas with all these temptations? One possible reason is that such knowledge could potentially free us from death, and thus from the clutches of Yama, forever. From the deity's perspective, that would be bad for business. But several commentators on this exchange suggest that Yama is actually testing Naciketas (as all Indian gurus would do to their prospective students) to see if the boy, despite his young age, is mature enough to receive the teaching. It's obvious from his responses to the increasingly alluring temptations that he is, and so Yama, praising Naciketas as "steadfast in truth" and wishing "May we find another questioner like you!" (2.9), begins the teaching on the "yoga of the inner Self" (adhyatma yoga) (2.12).

The chariot parable comes near the beginning of chapter 3. In it the chariot stands for the physical body and the rebellious horses are its senses, the chariot owner is the Self, and the charioteer and reins are two aspects of consciousness (citta), respectively, the intellect (buddhi) or "higher mind," the source of all wisdom, and the "lower mind" (manas), whose role is to mediate between the senses and buddhi.

The parable uses this simple set-up to contrast the life of an average person with that of a yogi. The former, whose consciousness is "undisciplined" (3.5) and without understanding, is at the mercy of its untamed "horses," the senses. The result is that the buddhi is unable to control the senses no matter how hard he pulls on the "reins" of manas, and hollers "Whoa!" We all probably know someone like this (and may in all honesty be one ourselves). Vyasa (see Chapter 4), Patanjali's oldest surviving commentator, calls such a mind kshipta, "scattered, distracted," and vikshipta, "agitated, bewildered."

Conversely the yogi's consciousness, which is well disciplined and steeped in understanding, has a firm "rein" on the "horses." This buddhi and manas then fulfill their proper roles, and the chariot with the Self onboard is successfully steered toward that ultimate of the yoga of the inner Self, self-understand and self-completion.

The "method" of course will vary according to the teaching of the school, though there may be more than one favored method in any one school. So, for example, the method most closely associated with Classical Yoga, the subject of Chapter 4, is the "eight-limb" or "step" (*ashta anga*) course of practice. But there's a second practice in the text that's often given short shrift or overlooked entirely. It's called kriya yoga, the yoga of "[ritual] action" (see YS 2.1–3). Both of these methods stand in sharp contrast, for example, to Hatha Yoga's focus on awakening the "sleeping serpent," the mysterious transformative force latent in each of us known as kundalini. We'll return to this in Chapter 5.

Our second misconception involves the meaning of the word "union." A quick check of the word in a dictionary reminds us that in order to have any union at all, we need at least two "things." When it comes to yoga, almost every major school agrees (with the notable exception of Classical Yoga, see Chapter 3) that these two things are our essential Self (what Mr. Iyengar calls our "individual soul") and the cosmic Self (Mr. Iyengar's "Universal Spirit"), often translated as "God."

Now it's quite understandable that we should speak of these two Selves as being separate from each other, because that's how we unconsciously experience the people and things in our world. From my point of view, for example, the elusive character named "Richard Rosen" is "in here," neatly packaged in this mortal frame (at least for the time being), while everyone and everything else—what we might call "not-Richard Rosen"—is "out there," divided from me by a seemingly unbridgeable gulf that isolates me in my own little patch of the world. A similar experience is true, I assume, for you.

But according to yoga, there's a problem with this way of seeing the world. While we may accept that we need two "things" to have a union, one of yoga's central tenets is that everything that exists, all "two-ness" or apparent diversity, can ultimately be resolved into a pre-existing unity or Oneness (usually spelled with a capital *O* to emphasize its all-inclusiveness). Most yoga schools are philosophically based on *monism*, which my dictionary defines as the "view that reality is one unitary organic whole with no independent parts." The famous "great saying" (*maha vakya*) of the *Chandogya Upanishad* (6.8.7)—*tat tvam asi*—affirms this view: "that" (*tat*), the *Brahman* or the cosmic Self, "is the same as" (*asi*) "you" (*tvam*), the essential Self.

From yoga's perspective, then, all separateness is, at best, a convenient way for us to manage the everyday business of encountering and navigating through the "not-me"; at worst, this separateness is an illusion based on our own mistaken perceptions (*avidya*), and the cause of an unremitting existential alienation and suffering.

BRAHMIN, BRAHMA, AND BRAHMAN

What's the difference between Brahmana, Brahma, and Brahman? These words are all related to each other through the root *brih*, "to increase, expand."

The word *Brahmana* has two general applications. First, it designates a collection of commentaries attached to the four foundation texts of the Vedic corpus—the Rig, Sama, Yajur, and Atharva Vedas (see Chapter 3). Second, Brahmana names Hinduism's priestly caste (which produced the Brahmana commentaries and so gave the texts their collective title), as well as the individuals who belong to this caste by birthright. But in the literature, we rarely see the word *Brahmana* used in this second way; instead, it's typically anglicized to *Brahmin*. One source claims the change was made to distinguish secularly employed Brahmanas from their priestly counterparts.[8]

Brahma (with a long final "a" and so pronounced bruh-MAH), a singular masculine noun, is the name of the creator god of Hinduism's holy trinity (*trimurti*). Alain Danielou renders the Sanskrit into English as "Immense-Being." The other two gods are Vishnu (the "all-pervader"), who sustains, and Shiva ("auspicious, benevolent"), who reabsorbs the universe at the end of its mind-bendingly long life cycle.

Finally there's Brahman, a singular neuter noun, which Dr. Feuerstein translates (based on the meaning of its root, *brih*) as "vast expanse" but which more often than not appears in English as the "Absolute." It's difficult to describe exactly who or what Brahman is because it transcends everything imaginable. As it's written in the *Taittiriya Upanishad* (2.9): "Before they reach it [Brahman], words turn back, / together with the mind. . . ." Suffice it to say that Brahman is the world-ground, on which everything that exists is founded and sustained, and to which it all ultimately returns.

Revelation

With this in mind, let's return to the question with which we began this discussion: What do we mean by yoga as "union"? We naturally assume that it means the joining (or perhaps rejoining), through the practice of yoga, of the two separate selves, the atman and the brahman. This is, as we have seen, a potentially grievous misconception, since the presumption of separateness itself is a root cause of suffering. In fact, yoga doesn't *effect* a union at all—it can't, because in the all-inclusive Oneness of the universe there aren't in reality two "things" to join. What yoga does instead is *reveal* to us that this "union," which we were so diligently hunting for through our practice, was right in front of our noses all along, hidden in plain sight.

Un-join

I saved my comments on the third misconception of "yoga means union" for last because I anticipate it'll generate the most controversy. I want to preface what follows then by saying that the opinions expressed are mine alone, that none of my teachers necessarily agree with me (in fact, I can think of a few who, if they bother to read this book at all, will likely disown me), and that I mean no harm to anyone's cherished beliefs.

I noted earlier that *most* yoga schools are "philosophically based on what's called *monism*." There is one prominent exception, the school of Classical Yoga (CY), which is philosophically based on *dualism*, the "belief that everything has two opposite parts or principles." The teachings of this school are outlined in the well-known if bare-boned *Yoga Sutra*, compiled sometime between 200 B.C.E and 400 C.E. (the dating is contested) by someone named, or at least calling himself, Patanjali. All of this will be covered in much greater detail in Chapter 4.

For now, let it be understood that when it comes to Classical Yoga, yoga *does not* mean union. Anyway Classical Yoga isn't about union at all; in fact it's just the opposite. Nor is it concerned with "enlightenment" per se. The entire thrust of practice in Classical Yoga is the complete and lasting escape from future existential suffering by gradually paring away the source of that suffering: all the false or mistaken identifications of the Self with matter. Thus, it's really more accurate to call the goal of Classical Yoga "dis-union" (*viyoga*), which is accomplished through intensive meditation. What actually gets freed isn't the Self, which is eternally free and so never bound, but a small bit of matter—formerly known as "my body-mind"—which is returned (or recycled) to the cosmic matrix (*pradhana*).

In support of this proposal I call on a pair of respected scholars. Professor Gerald Larson, who specializes in both Indian culture and religious studies, points out that the Sanskrit word "yoga" has two different roots, one meaning the familiar "yoke-join," the other meaning "in the sense of samadhi," a word we'll come across every now and then in this book. Samadhi, literally "putting together," is usually the last stage in a very intense process of meditation. To reach this rarified condition the meditator must use her consciousness to penetrate the essence of the object of her meditation, bypassing all of its superficial exterior qualities, so that she's "put together" with that object and comes to know its essence from the "inside out." (There's also a third *yuj* root, meaning "judicious control," though the "yoke-join" root seems to be the oldest—the other two being later derivatives.) Professor Larson writes that in the tradition of Classical Yoga, the word "yoga" is "seldom used in the sense of 'yoke,' 'join,' or 'union' as is sometimes claimed in popular accounts of Yoga. The term refers, rather, to concentration and is most easily understood in the *Yoga Sutras* . . . simply as 'disciplined meditation' in regard to the various states of awareness."[9]

Our other scholar is Edwin Bryant, a professor of Indian religion at Rutgers University. With respect to "union," he writes that the word is "best avoided" in discussions of the *Yoga Sutra* since the goal of yoga, as described in that work, is "not to join, but the opposite: to unjoin."

Bryant endorses a different translation of "yoga" altogether: For the traditional commentators of the *Yoga Sutras,* he writes, yoga means a fully concentrated mind.[10]

>> *The other day while reading a book about yoga, I came across a reference to the "science" of yoga. Surely yoga isn't a "science" like physics or botany, is it?*

> Where there is a "technique," there is science. Yoga has its own technique of physiological, psychological and supramental well-being of man. So it is a science. . . . Yoga is a science of character-building or right conduct.
>
> B. K. S. Iyengar, *Iyengar: His Life and Work* (1987), p. 189

> The science of Yoga gives a practical and scientifically prepared method of finding the truth in a religion.
>
> Swami Vishnudevananda, *The Complete Illustrated Book of Yoga* (1989), p. 5

Is yoga a science? The response we get depends in large part on whom we ask. Most mainstream scientists, whether they have spiritual inclinations or not, will probably answer, "No." Science is scientific, they say; it produces measurable results that can be re-created by anyone who follows the prescribed method or formula. For example, if I'm a chemist and I mix a specified amount of substance X with a specified amount of substance Y, under normal conditions, Z will be the result. No matter how many times I perform this same process, the result will always be Z, and the same goes for anyone else anywhere in the world—X plus Y will get Z.

Now consider the traditional teaching and practice of yoga. First of all, since each student had a close relationship with his or her teacher, the practice was devised to suit the character and abilities of the student; in other words, it was highly individualized. So while the goal or desired "result" of the practice was the same for all students, the means of getting there was, to a lesser or greater degree, different. If we imagine our practitioners as chemists, each one is mixing slightly different amounts of

X and Y to get to Z; moreover, no matter how many times they mix X and Y together, there's no guarantee that Z will ever be the result; and finally, to complete our analogy, Z is completely immeasurable!

But not everybody agrees with this assessment. Middle-of-the-roaders, those who straddle the worlds of both science and spirituality, insist there's really no contradiction between science and yoga. In their view, each functions in different (though intimately related) worlds—science, the material; yoga, the immaterial or spiritual. Each provides a slightly altered perspective of the same landscape, like two people standing a mile apart looking at the same mountain.

Then there are those who believe that the more that modern science advances, the more it affirms the ancient teachings of yoga.

So who's right? Is yoga a science? Or maybe, is science a yoga?

Here's something to think about: the root of "science" is the Latin *scire*, "to know" (also the root of "conscience"), which is related to *scindere*, "to cut, divide." This etymology tells us two things about science. First and most obviously, scientists are mostly interested in acquiring concrete knowledge, particularly about a world they see as wholly material. In such a world, human consciousness is relegated to a peripheral role, dismissed (if acknowledged at all) as a mere by-product of matter.

Second, scientists often acquire this knowledge by cutting or splitting. They try to cut themselves off from their world, by stepping back and studying things objectively, minimizing any subjective involvement. The classical scientist assumes it's possible to separate what's "out there" entirely from what's "in here."

But with the development of "new physics" over the last few decades, this dualistic stance is harder to defend. About seventy-five years ago, physicist Werner Heisenberg (the 1932 Nobel laureate in physics) postulated that the supposedly objective observer couldn't help but influence, at least in a very small way, whatever he was observing. This implies that there's no such thing as outright objectivity, and that we unavoidably influence any dealings we have with the world.

Scientists will also literally cut whatever it is they're studying into smaller and smaller pieces for a closer look. Physicists, for example, do this with matter in their particle accelerators by smashing atoms into each other. This is part and parcel of the scientific method, in which scientists first gather data based on observation, use this data to draft a hypothesis, run and rerun experiments that either prove or disprove the hypothesis, and finally, if the experiments confirm the hypothesis, draw conclusions and devise grand theories or natural laws (which they can always modify or scrap entirely in the future, if new information surfaces).

So how does yoga stack up as a science? Yogis surely value knowledge as much as scientists, but the knowledge they value most concerns the immaterial Self. Despite their often undeserved reputation as ascetic world-renouncers, yogis have also accumulated an encyclopedic knowledge about the material world, from which they've developed an intricate model of nature—though with its oceans of milk and mountain range extending a couple of billion miles long. In the quest for the Self, yogis have traversed all the realms of our world, physical and subtle, leaving no stone unturned, and every school of yoga has developed its own unique "yoga-tific method," which in its formal structure and approach to practice is every bit as systematic and rational as science's approach to understanding the material world.

Because of the fragmented way that yoga practice is ordinarily taught in the West, students tend to miss or misunderstand the yoga-tific method behind the seeming yoga madness. In fact, for many hundreds of years yogis have occupied themselves with self-observation and meditative experimentation, the building and testing of hypotheses, and fine-tuning theories about the nature, the mind, and the Self. This was all performed in the research laboratory of the yogi's own body-mind, then rigorously scrutinized and evaluated by students in his own school, rival schools, or even hostile schools. If a practice was found effective, if its initial results could be repeated much of the time by others following the same procedure, then it was adopted and integrated into the general method. But if it was found wanting, it was revised for further review or dumped on the yoga rubbish heap.

So it's no exaggeration to say that our "mystical" yogis are just as practical as scientists. Remember that while there's pure or theoretical (as opposed to applied) science, there's no such thing as purely theoretical yoga. In yoga, *speculation* about the practice always follows from the day-to-day mule work of *doing* the practice. Svatmarama writes, in the *Hatha Yoga Pradipika*, that as long as your practice hasn't reached its fullest expression in "spontaneous meditation," merely talking about spiritual knowledge is only "indulging in hypocritical and deceitful prattle" (HYP 4.114).

Of course scientists make their observations *on* the world *in* the world and minimize as much as possible—or so they hope—the subjective element. They put their trust in the evidence of their five senses, which are frequently extended or amplified by one or another scientific doodads. If a scientist can't see, touch, taste, or get an accurate measurement of what he's observing, it simply doesn't exist. By contrast, yogis feel that the senses are inherently limited, no matter how refined or amplified they are by instrumentation. You can surely discover lots of useful information about the world through your senses, but you can't know what's most important—the Self—by relying on the senses alone.

If the senses are so limited, how then do the yogis get to the heart of the matter, the Self? We'll talk about this more in Chapter 4. For now I'll remind you about the earlier discussion on samadhi, in which the meditator assimilates the object of meditation directly into her consciousness. Such "putting together" is no longer dependent on the senses to know the things of the world of matter.

So is yoga a science? There are obvious parallels between the methods of the scientist and the yogi, and both, in their own way, are searching for the truth at the heart of the world. But scientists seek knowledge that reveals and transforms the world; their own inner transformation is an afterthought (though they may be profoundly affected by their work). Yogis, on the other hand, while not indifferent to the world, seek only that knowledge that reveals the essential truth behind reality.

The answer to our question then is, most definitively, it all depends. If we interpret *scire*, "to know," in a strictly Western sense, then, no, yoga isn't truly a science. But if we allow ourselves to expand the territorial limits of this "knowing" to include the subtle and spiritual provinces—as the yogis do—then yoga is the supreme science, the science of all sciences.

» *Is yoga a religion?*

Yoga is not a religion . . . [It is] a method of physical and psychic culture. You may be a Christian, a Buddhist, a Moslem, or a Hindu, and yet a student of Yoga. You may also be an atheist. If you are, and you follow the Yoga path seriously, you will probably feel impelled to establish a new religion.

> F. YEATS-BROWN, *Yoga Explained: A Simple Approach*
> *to a Fuller and Richer Life* (1937), pp. 7–8

It [yoga] is non-sectarian and non-religious. It respects all religions and philosophies....

> SRI DEVA RAM SUKUL, *Yoga and Self-culture* (1947), p. 18

No one ... has to give up his devotion to Jesus if he walks on the path of the living [yoga] Masters. By this path, in fact, he becomes a better Christian. . . . The Masters do not establish new creeds or churches, and are friendly toward all existing religions.

> JOSEPH LEEMING, *Yoga and the Bible* (1963), p. 24

Yoga has no theology and ... does not mention God or in any way define him. It is a method, a system inevitably leading to religion and a religious outlook, as a ladder leads to an upper floor, but is not itself concerned with what is found on that upper floor.

> LAURENCE BENDIT, *Self Knowledge:*
> *A Yoga for the West* (1967), p. 4

It's common to mistake Yoga for a religion. . . . It is a system of philosophy and psychology rather than a religion.

> JOY HERRICK (with Nancy Schraffenberger), *Something's*
> *Got to Help—And Yoga Can* (1974), pp. 34–35

In all my thirty-six years as a yoga student and twenty-nine as a teacher, I can't honestly remember anyone ever asking this question. Yet several of my yoga-teacher friends assure me that they encounter it regularly. They tell me they hear it most frequently from new students, who may be worried that yoga is a wolf in sheep's clothing (the "wolf" being Hinduism). Some students fear that something sinister is lurking behind modern yoga's welcoming, come-one-come-all public persona—if they're not careful, soon enough they'll be donning robes and booking a flight for India. And should yoga lead them away from their own faith, the consequences would be catastrophic, not only in this life but especially the next.

Most of us aren't aware that Christians, for example, have been proselytizing in India since perhaps as early as the first century C.E. They've been hard at work trying to get Hindus to do exactly what many Christians fear yoga is trying to do to us—that is, convert them to their side. How have they done? A head count in 2011 found almost twenty-eight million Indian Christians, a pretty significant number, though when compared with India's total population of over 1.2 billion, it's a drop in the bucket.

So today the Christians in this country would seem to be confronted by an alien intruder from the very country they've been intruding in for centuries—a rather ironic reversal. As the saying goes, "Turnabout is fair play." Yogis, however, aren't actively trying to lure Westerners away from their faith. And not all religious leaders in the West share the same concern for yoga. Some are perfectly comfortable with their flock practicing yoga, without any caveats; others are fine with it as long as yoga classes are strictly for stretching and strengthening—as soon as the teacher starts OM-ing, the faithful are advised to head immediately for the nearest exit and, as Bob Dylan said, don't look back. Some of the more conservative religious groups, however, absolutely don't want their followers to have anything to do with yoga, imagining it to be a ticket to ride to eternal damnation.

Is any of this *Sturm und Drang* over yoga justified? Is yoga a religion? Naturally I'm biased, but the short answer is emphatically "NO!" Yoga isn't a religion, at least *not in the way it's generally taught in the West.* (Some yoga purists maintain that not only is Western yoga not a religion, it is not even yoga.) While there are indeed historical links between Hinduism and certain traditional schools of yoga, and while these links may yet survive in some form in *modern* yoga (see Chapter 5 on the difference between traditional and modern yoga), the connections are few and far between. For the vast majority of yoga students in the West, yoga has little to do with religion and everything to do with physical exercise, stress reduction, and basic self-healing. In no way does this threaten anyone's faith.

What about the religious trappings we see at most yoga schools—the serene Buddha statues, the OM symbols, the twanging sitar music? All of these are employed to create a "yogic mood," to prepare students to jump around or lay around and everything in between. They have nothing to do with religion.

Yoga teachers and yoga proponents are usually anxious to counter any suggestion that yoga is a religion, and there are two ways they typically go about this. The first is a flat-out denial: yoga is *not* a religion, period. I must have read this claim in at least fifteen books on my shelves, though none of these teachers could explain precisely how yoga is a "system" rather than a religion. Indeed, they seemed almost to protest too much, and in this way to contradict the very message they were trying so hard to affirm.

The second approach is simply to admit up front that, well, yeah, okay, yoga does have some religious associations. But the argument continues on two fronts:

1. These associations are ideas or behavioral injunctions that all religions will more or less agree with. For example, Christians and Jews will feel right at home with the behavioral injunctions, *which echo the Ten Commandments*: do not kill (*ahimsa*), always tell the truth (*satya*), do not steal (*asteya*), and don't be greedy (*aparigraha*). The *niyamas* (observances) also include values common to many faiths; purity (*santosha*) and scriptural study (*svadhyaya*) come immediately to mind (for more discussion of the *yamas* and *niyamas*, see Chapter 4).

2. These religious associations—which do include some beliefs at odds with Western faiths, such as *karma* and rebirth—aren't crucial to gaining the ultimate goal of the practice: to "know ourselves more profoundly and make sense of the world in which we live."[11]

So why do we resist labeling yoga a religion? I can think of two possible reasons, one altruistic, the other less so. First, as teachers we're well aware of the many benefits of a regular yoga practice, and we're eager to share these benefits with others. That's what we do; that's part of our passion for teaching. If people become convinced that yoga is a religion, they stay away from the practice, which would make us teachers very sad.

The second reason is, frankly, financial. We teachers, most of us anyway, make all or a large chunk of our living from teaching yoga, so fewer students will at some point affect the bottom line.

>> *I was watching a documentary on yoga and one teacher after another stated that yoga was five thousand years old. Where does this number come from?*

That these pre-Aryan people practiced a form of physical Yoga is indicated by the fact that certain seals were found during excavations carried out at the sites of Mohenjo-daro and Harappa. . . . The seals found there show a figure sitting in a Yoga position.

WILLIAM ZORN, *True Yoga* (1965), p. x

The earliest archaeological evidence for the practice of Yoga is afforded by some small figures of men in the posture of yogic meditation excavated in the Indus valley. They date from at least 3000 B.C.

HARI PRASAD SHASTRI, *Yoga* (1957), p. 13

In Asia . . . this secret knowledge of the human soul has been handed down from one generation to the next without a break for over six thousand years.

SELVARAJAN YESUDIAN and ELIZABETH HATCH,
Raja Yoga (1956), p. 38

Sometime in the 1820s, James Lewis (1800–1853), a soldier in the army of the British East India Company stationed at Agra, decided to prematurely end his military service—in other words, he deserted. Assuming the identity of an American from Kentucky named Charles Masson, he turned his back on his employer and headed west across the Punjab, a vast region that today spreads across northwestern India and northeastern Pakistan.

One day, in the valley of the Indus River, near the village of Harappa, he stumbled upon a long abandoned "ruinous brick castle," as he described it, surrounded by the fragmentary remains of buildings. Lewis/Masson learned that according to local tradition, this was once the site of a great city, "destroyed by a particular visitation of Providence, brought down by the lust and crimes of the sovereign." He was the first European to visit this place, but his stay turned out to be very brief. Later that evening, his party was assaulted by swarms of "makkahs," stinging gnats, which drove their horses frantic and forced the group to decamp and march throughout the night.[12] After several years on the lam and enough adventure to satisfy even Indiana Jones, Lewis/Masson, pardoned for his desertion, settled down and made a name for himself as an archaeologist and coin collector.

Harappa wasn't nearly as fortunate in its next encounter with the British. In 1856, railroad engineers carted off its brick ruins and crushed them into small stones to use as ballast for the tracks they were laying through the area. So the walls of Harappa, one of the oldest and largest of all Bronze Age cities—at its height its population was estimated at 23,000, making it a veritable New York City of its time—came tumbling down to line the beds of the Sind and Punjab Railway.

It took twenty years for the British to figure out that they'd dismantled an important archaeological site, and then another fifty or so before excavation began in what was left of Harappa. In the meantime, dozens of other sites were discovered throughout the Indus valley, revealing a far-flung civilization that began around 2600 B.C.E., then mysteriously disappeared about seven hundred years later. Most authorities fix the blame on a sudden, disastrous change of the river's course, depriving the cities along its banks of their water supply and putting a serious dent in agriculture and trade. But Indus expert Gregory Possehl asserts that the river's shift "doesn't explain the collapse of the entire . . . civilization." Throughout the valley, he says, an evolving culture reached "some kind of obvious archaeological fruition about 1900 B.C.E.," but what drove that, "nobody knows."[13]

In 1911, an Indian archaeologist found the remains of an even larger urban center, where the population was thought to exceed 30,000, a few hundred miles south of Harappa. Named Mohenjo Daro, the "Mound of the Dead" (its original name is unknown), digs there turned up a wealth of artifacts, including statues, tools, jewelry, toys, and small, carved soapstone seals. These seals had a variety of uses, most commonly to secure trading goods and identify the contents of the bundle and its owner. One of them, referred to in Zorn's quote above, is of particular interest to the yoga world. Slightly more than an inch square, it depicts a human-like figure, either horned or wearing a horned headdress, surrounded by six animals, which appear to be a rhino, an elephant, a buffalo, a tiger, and a pair of deer. Above the figure appear some characters or symbols, presumably an Indus valley script, though to this day they've never been deciphered. But what is most striking is the figure's sitting position, which looks for all the world like an asana, or yoga posture, today called Bound Angle (*baddha kona*). Sir John Marshall, then director-general of the Archaeological Survey of India and the leader of the late-1920s excavating team that uncovered the piece, named the figure Pashupati, the "lord" (*pati*) of "beasts" (*pashu*).

Now there's more to this appellation than meets the eye. Pashupati is a nickname of the Vedic god Rudra ("Howler"), who in later times transmogrifies into Shiva, one-third of the Hindu trinity and the divine progenitor and patron saint of Hatha Yoga. By assigning the figure the name Pashupati, Marshall seemed to imply that it represented an early form of Rudra/Shiva, sitting placidly amid his beastly posse, practicing yoga. Marshall's opinion carried great weight, and over the years other experts, among them German Indologist Heinrich Zimmer and American teacher and author David Frawley (now known as Pandit Vamadeva Shastri), climbed aboard the Pashupati bandwagon.

It was thus settled, with the backing of these powerful voices, that yoga began in the Indus valley, giving rise to the now familiar claim that the tradition is five thousand years old—although that estimate represents a generous rounding-up because Mohenjo Daro was established no earlier than around 2600 B.C.E., or 4,600 years ago.

But hold your rhinos, not all the experts are convinced by Marshall's call. Gavin Flood, professor of Hindu studies and comparative religion at Oxford, presents an entirely different perspective. To his way of thinking, it's "not clear from the seals that the . . . figure is seated in a yogic posture." In India 4,600 years ago, *everybody* sat on the ground as a matter of course, as many Indians still do today; so while the posture *could* be an asana, it ain't necessarily so. Flood refers to Finnish Indologist Asko Parpola, who has "convincingly suggested" that the figure isn't even a human, but is in fact a "seated bull."[14]

Flood is supported, among many others, by David Gordon White, professor of comparative religion at the University of California, Santa Barbara. Anyone hoping to reconstruct the history of yoga, White writes, "must resist the temptation of projecting modernist constructions . . . onto the past." Like Flood, White insists that the figure's identity "is open to question," and without more information, to identify the figure as a yogi is "therefore abusive."¹⁵ Now "abusive" may be a bit strong here, but you get the idea. We can readily accept that *some* yoga-like exercises *may* have existed in incipient forms in 2600 B.C.E., but the answers to exactly how and to what end they were performed are probably forever buried under the weight of fifty centuries.

But if we reject Marshall's idea about the Mohenjo Daro seal, or at least suspend judgment until more evidence comes in, we are brought once more to the question: How old is yoga? Nobody knows for sure. We *can* say, however, that yoga is *at least* as old as its first concrete mention as a practice, about 2,500 years ago in the *Katha Upanishad* listed below. Without question, yoga has existed as an oral tradition passed along from teacher to student for many hundreds of years. But more than 2,500 years? We can't say for sure.

> When the five knowings cease,
> Together with the mind,
> And intelligence does not stir,
> They call that the highest bourne.
>
> This steadfast control of the senses
> Is known as "yoga"—
> Then one becomes undistracted:
> For yoga is the origin and the passing away.
>
> *Katha Upanishad* 6.10–11 (translation by
> Valerie Roebuck)

» *Who was the first yoga teacher?*

> The primeval Hiranyagarbha, and none else, is the promulgator of the Yoga system.
>
> *Mahabharata* 12.350

> Hiranyagarbha is the expounded of the Yoga Shasta and none else older than him.
>
> *Brihad Yogi Yajnavalkya Smṛti* 12.5

Who was the first yoga teacher? That all depends on what you mean by "first." There are at least two possible answers to this question: one is a teacher of divine origin, the other of human origin. As it happens, both are named Hiranyagarbha, which is typically rendered into English as Golden Womb (*hiranya*, "gold," and *garbha*, "womb, embryo, fetus, child"), though we also find it as Golden Embryo, Golden Child, Golden Egg, or Golden Germ.

The earliest mention of the divine Hiranyagarbha, a Vedic god, is found in a *mantra* in the *Rig Veda* (see Chapter 3), the opening lines of which are remarkably similar to those of Genesis. The mantra praises him as the "Thread Self" (*sutra atman*), the Creator god who designs, builds, and then supports all that exists, on whom all things are strung like beads on a necklace:

> In the beginning the Golden Embryo arose. Once he was born, he was the one lord of creation. He held in place the earth and this sky. . . . He who gives life, who gives strength, whose command all the gods, his own, obey; his shadow is immortality—and death. (RV 10.121.1–2, translation by Wendy Doniger)

Swami Veda Bharati (writing under his former name, Usharbudh Arya) sees the deity Hiranyagarbha as the "cosmic mind," the "Teaching Spirit of the Universe." This implies that he's not merely the *first* teacher of humankind, but the *only* teacher that ever has been or ever will be. Swami Veda Bharati explains that all "revelation is of the grace that flows from the Golden Womb into the minds of those in meditation," and this wisdom is then passed along from one generation of yogis to the next throughout the centuries.[16]

So much for the Vedic god Hiranyagarbha, whom we'll designate Hiranyagarbha A. Some scholars assert that the earliest yoga teacher was a flesh-and-blood Hiranyagarbha (hereafter known as Hiranyagarbha B) whose dates, life story, and writings are lost to history. If there was indeed such a person, we can safely assume that he preceded Patanjali, the presumed compiler of the *Yoga Sutra,* most likely by several hundred years. If we situate Patanjali at the earliest of his possible dates, around 200 to 300 C.E., then Hiranyagarbha B could not have lived much later than the beginning of the first millennium C.E., though possibly quite a bit before then.

In what way does Hiranyagarbha B earn consideration as "first teacher" of yoga? It seems there are a good number of scholars who believe that Hiranyagarbha B was the first to teach the material eventually gathered into the earliest (surviving) presentation of a yoga system, the *Yoga Sutra*. Such a stance naturally challenges the cherished beliefs of those who credit this text, and the honor of compiling it, to Patanjali.

Now it isn't front-page news that Patanjali neither fashioned the philosophy behind nor invented the practices outlined in the *Yoga Sutra*. (Dr. Feuerstein, however, would strongly disagree with at least part of this statement; he asserts that the "philosophically grounded Kriya-Yoga" of *Yoga Sutra* 2.1–3 was "originally developed" by Patanjali.[17]) Professor Edwin Bryant points out that Patanjali admits as much himself in the famous opening sutra (1.1), though you have to know a little Sanskrit to catch it. You might recall that the sutra reads: *atha yoga anushasanam,* which translates as, "Now, the teachings of yoga." The prefix *anu-*, writes Bryant, is the giveaway, since it "indicates the continuation of an activity denoted by the noun to which it is prefixed"—that noun being *shasanam,* "teachings."[18] In other words, Patanjali is stating right up front that the material he has assembled isn't his; rather, as Mircea Eliade writes, he's simply "publishing and correcting . . . the doctrinal and technical traditions of Yoga"[19] that were well known to Indian ascetics and mystics for ages but had not yet been organized.

Of the several speculations crediting Hiranyagarbha B as the source of Patanjali's teachings, the one that carries the most weight for me (since it's recognized by no less an authority than Edwin Bryant) draws on a book titled the *Collection of the Serpent of the Deep* (*Ahirbudhnya Samhita*), written about 1,500 years ago (and which I've not been able to find in English translation). In it Hiranyagarbha B is acknowledged as the author of two lost books, the *Compendium on Restriction* (*Nirodha Samhita*) and the *Compendium on Action* (*Karma Samhita*).

The *Compendium on Restriction* arouses the most interest, because of two suggestive associations. First, the word that Hiranyagarbha B uses in the title for "restriction," *nirodha,* shows up in *Yoga Sutra* 1.2: *yogash citta vṛtti nirodhah,* "yoga is the restriction of the fluctuations of consciousness" (translation by Georg Feuerstein). Second, and perhaps even more telling, this *Compendium* is also known as the *Yoga Anushasanam*, the "Exposition of Yoga." Yes, that's right, the wording is almost the same as that of *Yoga Sutra* 1.1 cited at the start of this chapter. (If we apply Bryant's analysis again to this appearance of *anushasanam*, it would seem to suggest that Hiranyagarbha B was, like Patanjali, picking up on earlier material not his own, further complicating matters.) All in all, concludes Bryant, the information garnered from the *Collection of the Serpent of the Deep* suggests that Patanjali did nothing more than preserve the "ancient formulation of the original philosophy ascribed to Hiranyagarbha."[20]

These parallels convince some scholars that remnants of a historical Hiranyagarbha's original teaching are preserved in Patanjali's book, and that Patanjali himself probably was a student of Hiranyagarbha's school. In the end, however, all such conjecture, however intriguing, remains completely unverifiable.

» *I was at a lecture recently and the speaker said something about the "yoga darshana." Can you explain what that is?*

The Sanskrit word *darshana* comes from the root *dṛsh,* which means "to see" or "look." A *darshana* then is a way of seeing or looking—that is, a "viewpoint." The word is applied collectively to the six "orthodox" (*astika*, from *asti*, "there is," i.e., God) schools of Hinduism, the "six viewpoints" (*shad darshana*) that accept, or at least claim to accept, Vedic authority. They're called viewpoints because each is supposed to provide a different perspective on the same Truth similar to six people standing at regular intervals around a house. No one of them can see the whole house at once, but if each contributes his or her perspective to the group, an accurate picture of the house will emerge. These schools are set up against the unorthodox (*nastika*, those that hold "there isn't," i.e., God) schools like Buddhism and Jainism, which reject Vedic authority.

The six orthodox schools are traditionally paired. For our purposes, two pairs are most important: yoga (that is, Classical or Patanjali Yoga, based on the YS) and *samkhya* ("Enumeration"), and the two *mimamsa*

("Investigations"), the *purva* ("Earlier"), and *uttara* ("Later"), the latter of which is better known to the world as Vedanta (which we'll cover in Chapter 3). The teaching of each of these schools is outlined in texts written in the terse *sutra* style, the best known of which is the *Yoga Sutra*, the subject of Chapter 4.

The oldest of these viewpoints is Yoga's philosophical partner, Enumeration, which is something of an odd duck in the history of Indian thought, though its teaching has had a distinct influence on Hindu philosophy. The name "Enumeration" refers to the practice fundamental to this school, the enumeration or counting out of the principles (*tattva*) of nature. These principles evolve from the subtlest to the most concrete to create both the outer world of people and things, and the inner world of the mind. According to Enumeration, our mind is a material process—subtle to be sure, but material nonetheless. When we perceive, for example, a seat with four legs and a back, our consciousness (citta), which Classical Yoga conceives of as a very subtle material process, assumes the shape of this object, which we then label "chair."

Even odder than this, it seems to me, is Enumeration's proposal that all of nature is radically separate from the Self, a position known as dualism (which we can contrast with Vedanta's monism, discussed in Chapter 3). How it is possible for the latter to hook up with the former and then mistakenly identify with it is never explained (we'll come back to this question of the Self's misidentification with nature in Chapter 4). Each Self in turn is radically separate from all other Selves. This dualism is assumed by Classical Yoga as well, though there are several commentators who cast (or try to cast) the school in a monistic, Vedantic light.

One final note about Enumeration: it's an atheistic system. In other words it admits no God, considering such an entity unnecessary. Nature or the world is eternal, it has no beginning or end, it just keeps going and going and going, a wind-up toy with no innate intelligence.

TWO MORE DARSHANAS

Just in case you're interested, the other two viewpoints are called Method or Rule (*nyaya*) and Distinction (*vaisheshika*). Dr. Feuerstein explains that the former "seeks to ascertain truth by means of correct logical procedures of rules,"[21] and the latter "offers an approach to liberation through rational understanding of the categories of existence."[22] You needn't worry too much about either of these schools.

YOGA STORY

Samrambha Yoga: The Yoga of Fury

Our story opens with a brave and powerful but extremely impious king named Golden Clothes (*hiranyaka shipu*). When his younger brother, Golden Eyes (*hiranya aksha*), is killed by Vishnu, Golden Clothes decides that he himself will kill Vishnu. He conceives of a plan to acquire magical powers by impressing Brahma with his asceticism, and, sure enough, after some time the deity appears and offers him one boon. Golden Clothes then asks that he should never be killed by a god, a man, or an animal. This works just fine until Golden Clothes persecutes his pious son Delight (*prahlada*) for praising Vishnu ("all-pervader"), whereupon Vishnu appears in the form of a man-lion (*nara simha*)—half-human, half-animal, a neat end-run around the magical protection—and Golden Clothes is torn to pieces.

Golden Clothes next incarnates as the ten-headed and twenty-armed demon Crying Cause (*ravana*), a powerful, evil tyrant, invulnerable to men and gods. His story is told in the *Ramayana*, India's other great epic (along with the *Mahabharata*) whose hero, Rama ("pleasing, beautiful"), is yet another incarnation of Vishnu. Enraged by Rama's wars against his demons, Ravana kidnaps Rama's wife, Sita ("furrow"). This story ends much the same: once again, Vishnu—in the form of Rama, the half-human and half-god—kills Golden Clothes (in the form of Crying Cause).

Though you would think by now he might have learned an important lesson, our anti-hero reincarnates once again as an impious king, this time named Child Protector (*shishupala*). Needless to say, his hatred of Vishnu knows no bounds—a hatred which is further exacerbated when Vishnu, in the form of *his* latest incarnation, Krishna, kidnaps Child Protector's bride-to-be, Gold Adorned (*rukmini*), on their wedding day.

While attending a ritual sacrifice at which Krishna is also present, Child Protector calls him a fool and a low-class cowherd, among other incendiary names. A fight between the two inevitably ensues, and—you guessed it—Vishnu (now Krishna) goes 3-0 against Golden Clothes (now Child Protector), cutting off his head with a mighty heave of his discus. Because Golden Clothes' hatred of Vishnu is so complete, so all-consuming—such that it should cause his mind to be focused wholly upon the god throughout three lifetimes—it earns him a merit equivalent to that of a yogi engaged in intense meditation, and after his death Golden Clothes is united with Vishnu, "for the lord bestows a heavenly and exalted station even upon those whom he slays in his displeasure."[23] So ends the tale of a very exclusive school of yoga, called Samrambha Yoga, the yoga of "anger, fury, wrath," and its one and only adherent.

» *What is a guru?*

> Although many of the yoga traditions have textual foundations, the real foundation of the teaching of yoga is the guru. The practice of yoga is not traditionally learned from books, but from personal instruction.
>
> KNUT JACOBSEN, "Introduction: Yoga Traditions," in *Theory and Practice of Yoga*, Knut Jacobsen, ed. (2008), p. 22

> The master embodies Life, knows the truth, and leads on the Way that brings truth to form.
>
> KARLFRIED GRAF DÜRCKHEIM, *The Call for the Master* (1986), p. 39

The Sanskrit word *guru* is used rather loosely nowadays in the West to designate a "mentor" or an "expert" in a particular field or endeavor. We also see it appear in names for everything from bicycles to energy drinks, from apps for buying used cars to travel websites. But in ancient India the title *guru* wasn't handed out willy-nilly; instead, it was strictly reserved for a special type of spiritual teacher revered as God incarnate.

Like many of the words in the yoga lexicon, *guru* has a figurative or folk interpretation to go along with its dictionary meaning (in fact *guru* has four such interpretations, as we'll soon see). The dictionary defines *guru* as "heavy" (as well as "venerable"), which suggests that, as a bearer of liberating wisdom, a guru carries great weight.

While the dictionary tells us something about the guru's spiritual significance, folk interpretations riff on his function and nature. Four of these can be found in the *Song of the Guru* (*Guru Gita*), a text dedicated, as the title suggests, to all things *guru*. The "song" is a small part of the sprawling *Skanda Purana*, which may date to around 600 c.e.

How are these interpretations arrived at? First, the word *guru* is divided into its constituent syllables, *gu* and *ru*. Then each syllable is assigned one or more meanings, which are usually related (we'll see this same process applied to *hatha* in Chapter 5). What does the text reveal about the meanings hidden in *guru*? He's the one who:

> ...guides us from the "darkness" (*gu*) of self-ignorance to the "light" (*ru*) of self-realization (*Guru Gita*, 1.33; see also *Kularnava Tantra* 17.7).
>
> ...is "remover" (*ru*) of the "darkness" (*gu*) of self-ignorance (see also *Advaya Taraka Upanishad* 16).
>
> ...is totally free because he's beyond both the three "qualities" (*gunas*, see Chapter 4) of "nature" (*gu*) and all of its "forms" (*ru*) (*Guru Gita* 1.35).
>
> ...possesses the "supreme knowledge" (*ru*) that destroys all "illusion" (*gu*) (*Guru Gita* 1.36).

The syllable *gu* can also mean "cow" (though the more familiar spelling is *go*, as in *gomukhasana*, "cow face"). In this interpretation, the guru is pictured as feeding his student much like a mother cow feeds her calf.

What qualities might we look for when deciding whether or not someone is a true guru? The tenth-century *Kularnava Tantra* (13.57 ff.) lays out a laundry list of a true guru's characteristics, and suffice it to say that someone who embodies even half of these is a remarkable human being. One verse sums it up: "He who makes us know: 'I am the knower of the essence of all teachings, I am the core,' who is inseparable (from *Brahman*) and who is ever-pleased in heart'—he [who does that] is the Guru" (*Kularnava Tantra* 13.67).

Another text, the *Laws of Manu*, informs us in great detail how we should behave in the guru's presence. A guru is considered a deity, and a student is expected to treat him (and in ancient India it was almost invariably "him") with the kind of kowtowing reverence reserved in our time for rock stars and business moguls. Punishments for insulting the guru were severe to say the least, even extending beyond one's current incarnation. Speak ill of your guru, warns Manu (2.201), and in your next life you'll be reborn as a donkey. You'll wind up with a dog's life, literally, if you reproach the guru; a worm's life if you mooch off him; and an unspecified bug's life if you begrudge him.

Even so, it was understood then, as it still is today, that not all gurus were Dudley Do-Rights. The *Siddha Siddhanta Paddhati* advises us to abandon those gurus who delude us by means of their scriptural knowledge, who are ignorant, who don't tell the truth, or who are hypocritical (SSP 5.68–69). Certainly we can add to this that we should immediately reject a guru, or any teacher for that matter, who makes unreasonable financial demands, or who is verbally or physically abusive.

THREE TYPES OF *GURU*

Psychologist and Zen master Karlfried Graf Dürckheim (1896–1988), in his book *The Call for the Master* (1986), delineates three types of gurus, which he calls "masters": the archetypal or eternal master, the here-and-now master, and the inner master.

The first of these, as the name suggests, is a primal image that appears in consciousness in response to an encounter with "primal anguish." According to Dürckheim, this encounter might be triggered by some momentous event in our lives, or something as simple as a word or gesture. Whatever the cause, it shakes us out of our narrow, self-centered existence and wakes in us a "sudden and powerful longing for union with the Great Unknown,"[24] our true Self. The archetypal master then appears to help us find the way toward fulfilling this "promise felt within,"[25] the inkling we all have of our true Self waiting in the wings to be reclaimed. The here-and-now master is the living embodiment of the archetype. He or she exhibits a number of qualities, but of these, three are most essential: fullness, which manifests as "primal potency and strength"; order, which manifests as "special authority"; and unity, which is a "primal connection" with every living creature."[26] The final guru, the inner master, isn't a living person but an inner "authority," "forcing its way . . . toward self-realization in worldly form."[27]

Dürckheim goes on to list five things a guru or master does:

1. He/she teaches a specific doctrine that supports his/her teaching.
2. He/she interferes in the student's life; he/she "leads, corrects, and issues instructions."[28]
3. He/she radiates charisma, communicating with the student wordlessly and without doing anything. In this way, when the master is present, the "truth comes to light. Questions answer themselves before they are uttered. Obscurities vanish and facades collapse."[29]
4. He/she is an "example," who represents for the student the "looked-for, longed-for, ideal reality in human shape."[30]
5. He/she provides, when needed, a shock to the student's system, to "pull from underneath our feet the ground that prevents us from making contact with the true ground of existence."[31]

» *Do we really need a guru to practice yoga successfully?*

No guru, no book or scripture, can give you self-knowledge: it comes when you are aware of yourself in relationship. To be, is to be related; not to understand relationship is misery, strife. . . . Being confused in your relationship with people, with property, with ideas, you seek a guru. If he is a real guru, he will tell you to understand yourself. You are the source of all misunderstanding and confusion; and you can resolve that conflict only when you understand yourself in relationship.

JIDDU KRISHNAMURTI, *The First and Last Freedom* (2001), p. 135

In answer to this question, the yoga tradition responds with an emphatic "YES!" But not everyone agrees, especially the Indian "anti-guru" Jiddu Krishnamurti (1895–1986). I won't go into the details of his long and eventful life; it's easy enough to find out about him online. Be forewarned though that most of the websites you'll come across have nothing but effulgent praise for him and his teaching; however, if you dig a bit deeper, you'll find that he had, apparently, a side that was kept well hidden.

Krishnamurti's opinion, expressed in his usual uncompromising terms, is that we all tend to give gurus (and ourselves for that matter) far more credit than they (or we) deserve. At some critical juncture in our lives, we may discover a deep-seated urge to know the Truth. We then might turn to a guru for help, believing that on our own we're incapable of reaching the goal. In fact, Krishnamurti tells us, what we really unconsciously want from the guru is self-justification and self-gratification—in effect an *escape* from the Truth. He contends that no one, not even a guru, can bring us to the Truth; only we have that power.

Certainly we've seen plenty of instances over the past half-century of gurus run amok and disciples gone astray. We might take Krishnamurti's words as a caution, that we should closely examine our own motivations for seeking a guru and be alert for any signs of deceit or abuse. But why throw the guru out with the bathwater? It's possible, after all, that our motivations are proper and that the guru we approach wants only the best for the students he or she accepts.

>> *What are some common characteristics of the Indian guru?*

I've based my observations here on the biographies of numerous gurus, including Ramakrishna (1836–1886), Swami Vivekananda (1863–1902), Baba Premananda Bharati (1868–1914), Swami Rama Tirtha (1873–1906), Swami Sivananda (1887–1963), T. Krishnamacharya (1888–1989), Paramahamsa Yogananda (1893–1952), Swami Prabhavananda (1893–1976), J. Krishnamurti (1895–1986), Swami Omar (1895–1982), Swami Prabhupada (1896–1977), Shri Yogendra (1897–1989), Swami Muktananda (1908–1982), Swami Satchidananda (1914–2002), K. Pattabhi Jois (1915–2009), B. K. S. Iyengar (1918–2014), Maharishi Mahesh Yogi

(1918–2008), Swami Rama (1925–1996), Yogi Bajan (1929–2004), Bhagwan Shri Rajneesh (1931–1990), and Amrit Desai (1932–).

BIRTH

The future guru is invariably a male. His economic class varies: many come from well-to-do families; others may grow up in relative poverty, though most are born to a Brahmin family. He's often born at some astrologically propitious time, or in a spiritually significant place, or during a spiritually significant festival. Sometimes an astrologer or spiritual master predicts great things for him in the future.

CHILDHOOD

He's often unusually bright for his age, even debating with adults. Sometimes he's said to have psychic powers or visions, or demonstrates spiritual inclinations or flashes of illumination. He also sometimes displays heartwarming compassion for the poor and for animals. He often has a traditional spiritual upbringing, sometimes taught by his father from venerated texts like the *Rig Veda*. His mother is usually deeply religious.

TEEN YEARS

He's often an outstanding student at school. If he was born during the British rule of India, he might be educated in English at a Western-style school. (The one glaring exception to this is Krishnamurti, who was academically challenged and a poor student.) He might also display other remarkable talents or gifts, perhaps in singing, acting, athletic ability, or writing. As a result of his superior intellectual and/or artistic abilities, it's widely agreed among family and friends that he's destined for a successful career in the world. Indeed, the future guru might start out as a mathematics or philosophy professor, a doctor, or an engineer, though sometimes he may struggle financially. Sometimes a parent dies when the future guru is young or a wife dies early on in marriage, precipitating a spiritual crisis.

EARLY ADULTHOOD

He may work at some high-paying job but ultimately he will become dissatisfied by material life, and his spiritual longing will compel him to leave mundane life behind (Swami Rama Tirtha, for example, abandoned his wife and children). The future guru almost always first becomes the disciple of a guru, typically another man, though sometimes not (Krishnamurti had no guru; one of Ramakrishna's teachers was a female ascetic). He often meets his guru in a chance encounter and may immediately recognize and accept his guru, or he may go through a difficult period of doubt before committing to his teacher. The initiation process is usually a deeply transformative experience. Often the future guru is completely dedicated to his guru, but sometimes the relationship is rocky; the early difficult relationship between Krishnamacharya and Iyengar is one example, another is Vivekananda's initial ambivalence to Ramakrishna. There's often a period of months or even years spent alone, wandering in the "wilderness," whether in the Himalayas or across the length and breadth of India. This might be occasioned by a death in the family, or under the instructions of his guru. Sometimes he has surprisingly progressive ideas for his time and place (Shri Yogendra, e.g., favored female education), though he can also be a strict traditionalist (Krishnamacharya, e.g., at first refused to accept female students). He often has wealthy patrons, either a successful businessman or Indian royalty.

He might leave India for the West (though Krishnamacharya and Swami Sivananda did not). His reasons for such a trip might be several: He might be sent on a mission by his guru to spread some gospel to the world, either of Hinduism or some form of yoga, or his purpose might be to raise money for social causes, or he may simply heed a "call from within." His message is often well received in the West, at least initially. He frequently attracts well-to-do supporters who give him money and property, and he sometimes amasses a fortune himself. He establishes some kind of an ashram, organization, or institute, which grows and spreads across the region or country, or perhaps dies out after he leaves the United States (though he may not leave).

Sometimes he develops an innovative yoga practice that he synthesizes from various existing practices, though often he tries to associate his invention with traditional teachings to give them the appearance of ancient authority. If he returns to India, he might be welcomed as a conquering hero. He might end his life with a "miraculous" death, though his disciples don't call it "dying" but rather "entering *maha samadhi*" or "leaving his body." Sometimes something seemingly miraculous happens after his death (for example, his body doesn't decay).

» *What was a traditional yoga student like?*

> He who bestows the great lore... one should always betake to service under him, with superior wisdom. Whatever in this world, whether productive of happiness or misery or otherwise, is the mandate of the Guru, that the disciple should carry out with pleasure, without any scruple whatsoever.
>
> *Brahma Vidya Upanishad* 28

Yoga students today, for better or worse, bear little resemblance to their traditional predecessors, and I'm not talking just about the expensive clothes we wear and yoga mats we bring to class. Just about anyone can show up for a yoga class; when the class ends, everyone returns to going about their business. But in the old days yoga *was* a student's business, and he was held to extremely high standards of conduct and commitment. We can take as an example a list drawn from the *Kularnava Tantra* (13.23–30), which describes the characteristics of the kind of person, a thousand years ago, who might have attracted a guru's attention: the student would be pure, clean, truthful, diligent, heroic, thoughtful, trustworthy, honest, modest, enthusiastic, helpful, genial, celibate, and contented. Other lists describe even more admirable qualities: faith, veneration for the teacher, a moderate diet, desire to study the old texts, generosity, and most of all, an intense longing for liberation (*mumukshutvam*).

No offense to modern students, especially my own, but we'd all be hard pressed to get the nod from a traditional guru.

YOGA STORY

King "Great Chariot" (Brihadratha) and the Guru Shakayanya

A typical example of the great lengths to which disciples once went to impress a guru and win his favor is recounted in the *Maitri Upanishad* (1.2 ff.), from the third century B.C.E. The hero of the tale is King

Brihadratha, who was one day seized by a desire to leave behind the worldly life and take up the life of the spirit. He abdicated his throne and enacted a radical plan to obtain the favor of a guru. He "went forth into the forest" and for a thousand days he stood stock-still, "keeping his arms erect, looking up at the sun." The strategy proved successful. When the guru Shakayanya strolled by, he granted Brihadratha a single boon. (We might imagine that the king would have merited more than *one* boon, since after nearly three years in this position his arms were permanently stuck in place and he had lost his sight, but apparently Shakayanya was a tough customer.) "Be pleased to deliver me," Brihadratha pleaded. "In this cycle of existence I am like a frog in a waterless well. Sir, you are our way of escape."

2

PERFECTED
What Is Sanskrit?

samskṛta • put together, constructed, well or completely
formed, perfected; made ready, prepared, completed, fin-
ished; dressed, cooked (as food); purified, consecrated,
sanctified, hallowed, initiated; refined, adorned, orna-
mented, polished, highly elaborated (especially applied
to highly wrought speech, such as the Sanskrit language
as opposed to the vernaculars); a man of one of the three
classes who has been sanctified by the purificatory rites; a
learned man; a word formed according to accurate rules;
preparation or a prepared place, sacrifice; a sacred usage
or custom; the Sanskrit language . . .

From *A Sanskrit-English Dictionary* (1899),
by Monier Monier-Williams

MANY YEARS AGO AT THE outset of my yoga career, I decided
to teach myself Sanskrit. It turned out to be a bad idea, and, based on
my earlier failed attempts in high school to learn German and in college
to learn French, I (as the Beatles once sang) should have known better.
Several times over the next two decades I picked up the project of learning Sanskrit. Each time I began anew I promised myself that I wouldn't
give up until I'd reached a basic level of competence in Sanskrit—and
on every occasion I broke that promise and slunk off, my Sanskrit tail
between my legs.

Then about five years ago, I was offered the chance to join an informal weekly study group lead by a brilliant young Sanskritist who'd learned his business at Oxford. Our group of about fifteen started out, as these groups tend to, bright-eyed and bushy-tailed, buoyed by our teacher's promise that with just a half-hour of study each day, six days a week, we'd all be chattering away and gossiping in Sanskrit in no time at all. It didn't quite work out that way. At the end of eighteen months, on the eve of the teacher's departure for a yearlong sabbatical to India, there were just two of us left from the original group. And while I could stumble along through a text with the help of a dictionary and Sanskrit "cheat sheet," all of my gossiping was confined to English.

When the teacher left for India, I was determined to soldier on but knew I wouldn't go far on my own. So I hired a tutor, a scholar who had learned his Sanskrit in India and who lectured at the local school of higher learning, a place called the University of California, Berkeley. Once a week I climbed up into the Berkeley hills and sat for an hour in his living room, overlooking the campus and the campanile, working on translations of various texts. This went on for about two years, my daily study now extended from its original thirty minutes to around two hours. Finally, when I agreed to write this book, I had to stop my lessons, as my study time was now needed for research and worrying about deadlines.

This woeful tale probably doesn't spark in you an interest in learning Sanskrit, but let me assure you that for all its pull-out-your-hair-by-the-roots frustrating complexity, Sanskrit is a fascinating language. There are many things in my life that need doing that I don't look forward to, but my daily Sanskrit study wasn't one of them. I treated it as yoga for my brain, a practice that stretched and strengthened the synapses, improved my concentration, and taught me all about forbearance (*kshama*), persistence (*sagrada*), and most of all humility (*amanitva*). Beyond all this, Sanskrit opened a door to the old yoga texts and gave me an entirely new insight into their teachings. Reading these texts in their original language brings out subtleties inevitably lost in translation. For all its difficulties and sheer craziness, I love Sanskrit.

At first, however, I didn't think I'd include this chapter, believing it had only very limited appeal. But after talking with several of my students, who showed genuine interest when I described to them the chapter's outline, I changed my mind, so here it is. You should know that my intent isn't to teach you the language—I doubt I could even if I wanted to. Rather, my hope is to give you a basic understanding and some simple tools to work with so that as your yoga career progresses your encounters with Sanskrit will be enjoyable and profit you and your practice.

>> *I've been learning how to use a basic online Sanskrit-English dictionary. I tried to look up the word "Sanskrit," but I can't find it anywhere. How can it be that this word isn't in a Sanskrit dictionary?*

Suppose we wanted to look up the word "Sanskrit" in a Sanskrit-English dictionary. We'd go to the appropriate section and search…and search… and search some more. But no matter how much we searched, we'd never find it. How's that possible? Why isn't "Sanskrit" in the Sanskrit dictionary? Well, it's not there for the simple reason that "Sanskrit" isn't a Sanskrit word. It's a good example of "anglicization," that tendency we have to alter strange-sounding or strange-looking foreign words, to "English them up" so to speak, to make them easier for us to pronounce or spell.

The proper name for what we call Sanskrit is *saṃskṛta*. Here we see up-close-and-personal how anglicization works: the pinched-nose nasalization represented by the *-ṃ-* is converted to a more mellifluous *n*; the throat-choking *-skṛt-*, which neither looks nor sounds like English, is softened with an *i*, becoming the more English-friendly *-skrit-*; and the final *a*, which is inherent in the preceding *t* (see the following on the Sanskrit "alphabet"), is dropped as unneeded.

Even though *saṃskṛta* is the proper name of the language, we'll continue then to run with "Sanskrit" for the rest of this book. Take note that I capitalize the leading *s* of "Sanskrit," while I don't do the same for *saṃskṛta*. The reason for this is that formal Sanskrit, unlike English, hasn't any capital letters (what linguists call majuscules). So except for capitalizing book titles and the names of characters, like Patanjali (see Chapter 4) and Svatmarama (see Chapter 5), we'll stick to small letters (miniscules) when spelling Sanskrit words.

» What does "Sanskrit" mean?

Saṃskṛta is composed of two smaller words, *sam*, "together" (which further implies "union, thoroughness, intensity, completeness"), and *kṛta*, "done, made, accomplished" (but also "proper, good, cultivated"). As you can see from the dictionary entry that begins this chapter, the combination of these two simple words gives rise to a host of meanings. Not surprisingly then, there are several different opinions about which English word defines the language best. It appears that originally Sanskrit was no more than an adjective for what its speakers knew simply as the "language" (*bhasha*). According to the entry in the Anglo-Indian dictionary *Hobson-Jobson*,[1] the name Sanskrit wasn't widely used until British researchers began investigating the language in the late eighteenth century.

The different ways of defining "Sanskrit" each emphasize a different aspect or quality of the language. Swiss philologist Frederick Bodmer (1893–1955) renders Sanskrit as "arranged, ordered, correct," emphasizing its artificiality and "constructed" nature. He explains that as the language of the "priestly caste," along with "high-class secular literature," grammarians "drew up a code of correct usage" to preserve Sanskrit's "purity from contamination with low-brow idiom."[2]

This leads to another common definition, "refined" or "polished." In addition to suggesting that Sanskrit has been grammatically purified — the dross removed from the ore — these words have definite class connotations. In India, Sanskrit has always been spoken by the "refined" upper class (and this meant, for a good part of its history, that it was spoken almost exclusively by men). In this sense, Sanskrit is opposed to Prakrit (an anglicization of *prakṛta*), the collective name for the vernacular languages that were spoken by the hoi polloi. Prakrit means "natural" (in contrast to Sanskrit, which is "artificial"), but also, quite unfairly, "vulgar" and "unrefined."

Scholars and Sanskrit enthusiasts debate over which came first, Sanskrit or the Prakrits. The latter insist that Sanskrit is the "chicken" and all the Prakrits are her "eggs," the derivative tongues. At least one scholar agreed with this assessment. William Whitney (1827–1894), a well-respected nineteenth-century Sanskritist, described the Prakrits as "later and derived dialects" of Sanskrit.[3] Not so fast, counters Professor Wendy Doniger (b. 1940). She contends that it's just the other way around, that the vernacular languages are the "hen," while Sanskrit, the "refined, secondary revision, the artificial language" (as opposed to the naturally evolving Prakrits) is the "egg." It's only because Sanskrit was written down and preserved much earlier than the Prakrits, she explains, and so "won the race to the archives" that we imagine it to be the elder language.[4]

"Perfected" is a third common definition of Sanskrit. Present-day enthusiasts interpret it to mean that Sanskrit is the "perfect" language—an attractive selling point for those who might promote its teaching. At the outset though, according to German philologist and Orientalist Max Müller (1823–1900), the language made "fit for sacred purposes . . . the ancient idiom of the Vedas, was called Sanskrit, or the sacred language."[5]

» *Where does Sanskrit come from?*

There's no consensus on how many living languages there are in the world today. Estimates range from about five thousand to something over eight thousand—it all depends on how you define "living" and "language." Whatever the number is, these languages, like all living things, are divided into "families." Again there's no consensus on how many of these there are, but in the end it really doesn't matter because seventy-five percent of all living languages belong to just ten families. One of these is Proto-Indo-European (abbreviated PIE), which is the name that scholars have given to the reconstructed root language. They speculate that it was first spoken at least 5,500 years ago around the Caspian Sea in eastern Europe, and spread from there in all directions. Nowadays half the people in the world, including English speakers, speak a language that can be traced back to PIE.

PIE is itself subdivided into smaller families, one of which is the Indo-Aryan (or Indic), the eldest member of which is Vedic (often called Vedic Sanskrit). The emergence of Vedic is typically dated from about 1700 to 1200 B.C.E. As the name suggests, Vedic is the language of the Veda, the collection of Hindu holy books that are the subject of the next chapter. Vedic was superseded sometime around 400 B.C.E. by what's called

Classical Sanskrit, the Sanskrit we're familiar with through our yoga studies and classes.

The foregoing is what we might call the "academic" version of Sanskrit's origin, or what traditionalists would describe as "wrong." Sanskrit, according to their view, was taught to inspired sages by the deities at the start of the current world cycle. "Since the start of human civilization . . . people and the sages both spoke pure Sanskrit language." The traditionalists claim (without any concrete proof) there were public recitals of Hindu holy books as far back as 3072 B.C.E., more than five thousand years ago.[6]

>> *My teacher says that Sanskrit is the oldest language in the world and so by extension the "mother" of all languages. Then I read online that it's not even close to the oldest language, and that there are hundreds of languages that have no connection to Sanskrit whatsoever. What's the truth here?*

> Sanskrit . . . is considered to be the oldest language in the world, being at least 6,000 years old, and probably much older.
>
> ATMA INSTITUTE[7]

> Sanskrit is the Divine mother language of the world.
>
> THE VEDIC FOUNDATION, "Sanskrit: The Mother of All Languages"[8]

We're often assured by Sanskrit traditionalists that Sanskrit is the "oldest language in the world." If it's indeed the oldest, then it can't be an offspring of an even older predecessor. But scholars tell us that Sanskrit evolved out of Vedic, which in turn they trace back ultimately to PIE, which then assumes the mantle of "oldest language" (among, that is, the members of its family). When arguing Sanskrit's case, supporters ignore or deny the "parenthood" of PIE; in fact they might even insist this ancestral language never existed, that it's a "monstrous lie" fabricated by Western scholars. To them it's "quite evident" that Sanskrit is the "first and original language of the world," though I must say the proof they present to support this claim can be summed up as "because we say so." There are two problems with this position.

The first is that there are hundreds of languages in the world that decidedly aren't in any way related to Sanskrit, so Sanskrit can't be their "mother." Second, scholars estimate that human language first emerged around one hundred thousand years ago, and that all languages undergo a slow but steady evolution (though this isn't exactly true for Classical Sanskrit). This makes it impossible to definitively determine where one language ends and another begins. *All* languages then can be said to be equally old or equally young, and so the question of which is the oldest is meaningless.

But what if we revise the statement of the traditionalists—that Sanskrit is the "first and original language of the world"—to read more reasonably that Sanskrit is the oldest *surviving* language *still spoken today*. Extensive research turns up no agreement among the many language mavens, professional and amateur, contributing their two cents to this question. Vedic (and so the related language of Classical Sanskrit) is undeniably a strong contender for the "oldest" title, but no stronger, as it turns out, than Hebrew, Greek, Mandarin Chinese, or Tamil, which is spoken by more than seventy million people, mostly in southern India and Sri Lanka.

» *Is Sanskrit a dead language?*

This isn't, as you can imagine, a burning question in the everyday yoga community. But if you Google it you'll quickly find yourself engulfed in a worldwide controversy among Sanskrit scholars, educators, Indian nationalists and their detractors, as well as people who make some or all of their living selling Sanskrit courses and teaching materials. It's not possible for me to present the nuances of these arguments here; the conflicting opinions are just too many and convoluted to cover adequately in limited space. So let me just give a brief summary of the situation.

Scholars distinguish between languages that are living, dead, or extinct. A living language, as the name suggests, is a language in common use, spoken and written by living people, which changes over time to accommodate changes in the world it describes. Conversely, an extinct language is no longer spoken by anyone now alive, though scholars may be able to read and write it. A familiar example of this is the Old English of the epic poem *Beowulf*. A dead language inhabits the middle ground between living and extinct. While it might still be spoken by living people (who may or may not understand what they're saying), it's typically reserved for special occasions and is not in everyday use. A familiar example of this is Latin, the official language of the Catholic Church, which is used in their formal ceremonies and services, but is no longer a medium of casual conversation in the world at large.

The Indian yes-it's-alive camp points to a number of signs they interpret as proof positive that their opponents are, to put it mildly, not at all well informed: Sanskrit is one of twenty-two official languages in India; it's still taught in several prestigious universities; it has its own radio broadcasts and newspapers; contemporary Indian writers and poets still turn out books in Sanskrit and musicians still write and sing songs in the language; and there's reputedly a village in India where Sanskrit is spoken in everyday conversation (though it's not clear whether that means exclusively or frequently, and whether all villagers participate or only some).

Despite all this, the cold, hard numbers of a recent Indian survey tell us that just over 14,000 of its citizens say they speak Sanskrit as a first language, and fewer than 200,000 claim it as a second language, and that in the rest of the world there are only 16,000 speakers.[9] In a country whose population is now over 1.2 billion, these aren't exactly impressive numbers. Moreover, according to some academics, even these modest figures are suspect. People, it seems, tend to exaggerate their Sanskrit chops since it's considered a prestige language.

The no-it's-dead camp isn't as outspoken as its opponents, I assume because from its point of view, the answer to the question is such a slam dunk there's really nothing left to say. A respected and convincing advocate for this side is Sheldon Pollock, professor of South Asian studies at Columbia University and the general editor of the Clay Sanskrit Library, which now includes fifty-six volumes, covering Sanskrit drama, poetry, and novels, along with the two great national epics, the *Ramayana* and the *Mahabharata*; in other words, he's someone whose opinion about the state of Sanskrit today should be taken seriously (unless of course you don't happen to agree with him). In a long essay with the revealing title "The Death of Sanskrit," Professor Pollock argues that despite the enormous amount of time, effort, and money the Indian government has invested in supporting Sanskrit, while "feeding tubes and oxygen tanks may try to preserve the language in a state of quasi-animation . . . most observers would agree that, in some crucial way, Sanskrit is dead."[10]

These two camps represent the extremes of the Sanskrit living-or-dead controversy. There are, however, other possible answers, which have nothing to do with life or death. For example, Austrian Orientalist Maurice Winternitz (1863–1937) wrote in his *History of Indian Philosophy*:

> Sanskrit should never be spoken of as a "dead" language, rather as a "fettered" language, inasmuch as its natural development was checked, in that, through the rules of the grammarians, it was arrested at a certain stage. . . . What we call "Classical Sanskrit" means Panini's Sanskrit, that is, the Sanskrit which according to the rules of Panini's Grammar, is alone correct. In the "fetters" of this Grammar, however, the language still continued to live . . . [and] is not a "dead" language even to-day.[11]

PANINI

We might wonder about Herr Professor Winternitz's reference to Panini. What does a grilled sandwich have to do with Sanskrit? Well, this Panini (pronounced PAH-nee-nee) was a groundbreaking Indian Sanskrit grammarian, who might have lived in the sixth, fifth, or fourth century B.C.E., no one is exactly sure. His universally acclaimed grammar (which, like many ancient Indian texts, borrowed without attribution from earlier texts), consisting of nearly four thousand rules distributed among eight chapters, is rather unimaginatively titled *Eight Chapters (Ashtadhyayi)*. These rules were composed (either in writing or orally and then memorized, again no one is sure) in the very terse sutra style (see Chapter 4), each sutra consisting of no more than two or three words (the printed version of the text would likely cover no more than fifty pages). As is typical of this genre then, it's mostly incomprehensible without a commentary (compare the YS, see Chapter 4).

Practically everyone who chimes in on the *Eight Chapters* agrees that it's "one of the greatest intellectual achievements of any ancient civilization."[12] "Practically," though, doesn't include everybody. English Orientalist Henry Colebrooke (1765–1837), called the first great European Sanskrit scholar, complained that Panini made his head spin, and that in reading Panini he "wanders in an intricate maze," where the key keeps "slipping from his hand."[13]

Despite Colebrooke's reservations, Panini's work was so influential in India that no other grammarian dared challenge its basic premises. This essentially brought the natural development of Sanskrit to a screeching halt, and fixed it within certain artificial limits. While most languages usually get simpler over time, Sanskrit is stuck with a lot of rules that complicate its complications, making the language a tough nut to crack.

Professor Lakshmi Kanta Maitra turns the "dead" issue on its head. It's not Sanskrit that's dead, he charges, but the miscreants who make such a claim, because they're "dead to all sense of grandeur . . . dead to all that is great and rich in your own culture and civilization."[14]

Finally we have Sanskrit professor Robert Goldman, who rises above the fray completely by commenting that Sanskrit occupies a special niche among all world languages, being the only one that can't be labeled either "living" or "dead." He concludes that it's a "special, timeless language whose recitation, chanting, and even speaking are still much practiced and prized in India in certain contexts."[15]

» I'm interested in learning the Sanskrit alphabet. Can you tell me the most important things I might need to know about it?

If we open just about any Sanskrit primer to page 1, lesson 1, we'll find there an introduction to the "Sanskrit alphabet." We might also Google that term, and presto, in a third of a second, we're up to our ears in almost 280,000 results. There's only one problem: properly speaking, there's no such thing as the "Sanskrit alphabet."

Actually there are two problems. The first is that there isn't now, nor has there ever been, an "official" Sanskrit script. For many centuries, Sanskrit was written in the script of whatever happened to be the local vernacular (this is what's known as multiscriptism). It's only over the last hundred years or so, writes Professor Walter Maurer, that the tendency has become "more and more deeply rooted" to use a script named *nagari* (NAH-guh-ree) or *devanagari* (day-vuh-NAH-guh-ree) (some scholars date the beginning of Sanskrit's preference for *nagari* one or more centuries earlier). *Nagari*, which is the feminine form of *nagara*, "town born, spoken in town," is generally defined as "city-writing." This suggests that writing began in urban centers or towns, although Professor Müller cautions that the derivation from "town" is only speculation.[16] The second word, *devanagari*, relays the same message except that the "city" of origin is located in the heavenly realm populated by gods (*deva*). British scholar A. A. Macdonnell (1854–1930), writing at the beginning of the twentieth century, describes *devanagari* as a "term of late but obscure origin."[17]

These aren't the only interpretations of *nagari* and *devanagari*. Benjamin Walker cites unnamed scholars who assign *nagari*'s development to the "Nagas, an early Mongolian people of north-western India, since the script was also called Nagalipi, 'Naga-writing.'"[18]

Indian Sanskritist M. R. Kale, writing in the 1890s, speculated that the *deva* of *devanagari* (which literally means "to shine," and which is the root of the English "deity") referred to the supposedly fair-skinned emigrants (or as many would claim, invaders), the Aryans, who entered (or invaded) northern India from central Asia more than 3,700 years ago. He concluded that *devanagari* was a name for the Aryan (*deva*) settlements (*nagari*) in which Sanskrit was spoken. Kale's grammar is still available online, but his thoughts on the meaning of *devanagari* have been discredited by modern scholarship.

There's also a chicken-or-the-egg disagreement over which of the two names, *nagari* or *devanagari*, came first. Traditionalists champion the script's divine origin and so contend that *devanagari* is the correct name, while *nagari* is its shortened form. But most Western scholars, such as Professor Maurer, affirm the opposite, that *nagari* is the earlier name to which *deva* was prefixed much later.

Whatever the two words may mean, *nagari* has been the most frequently used of all the many scripts for writing Sanskrit books,[19] and as a result, it's now generally accepted as what most people call the "Sanskrit alphabet." But in fact, *nagari* and Sanskrit have what we might imagine as an "open relationship." There are a good number of modern Indian languages written in *nagari,* including Hindi, the country's official language, and even today Sanskrit books are occasionally printed in Bengali and Malayalam.

Now, with the understanding that Sanskrit has been and still is written in more than one script, we might accept *nagari* as Sanskrit's "official" alphabet, but to call it such perpetuates another misconception. Technically speaking, an alphabet consists of letters, like our Roman *a, b, c, d,* and so on. But only the thirteen *nagari* vowels are letters (or fourteen if we count the imaginary long *l*-vowel, more on this below). The thirty-three consonants are actually syllables, which Indian grammarians call "imperishable" (*akshara*), because unlike words that come and go, syllables are unchanging. When any one of the signs for these thirty-three consonants stands alone (that is, without being modified by any other vowel or consonant sign or signs), it's understood to be followed by an unwritten short *a* (there's also a long *ā,* more on this below). This *a* is always pronounced like the first and last letters of the English word "America" (that is, "uh"), the sound of which is technically known as a schwa (symbolized ə). So, for example, take the *nagari h.* Though it's represented by a single sign, we have to read or say it as if it were spelled *ha* (pronounced "huh"). In writing then, the word "hatha," which has five Roman letters, would need only two *nagari* characters, the *ha* and the *tha*, and neither of the *a*'s would be written (and the *th* is represented by just one character).

Since *nagari* is composed of both letters and syllables, it's not an alphabet but what's variously called a syllabic alphabet, an alpha-syllabary, or (my favorite) an abugida (from an Ethiopian name for Ge'ez writing, taken from four characters of that script, *a-bu-gi-da*).

» *Speaking of Sanskrit*

Before we proceed further, there are two words we should be clear about. The first is "translation," which is the rendering of one language into another, like Sanskrit into English. The second word, "transliteration," isn't as well known. It means to in some way represent or spell the characters of one script in those of another; for example, putting *nagari* characters into their Roman alphabet equivalent, a process that's sometimes called romanization.

Mispronunciation of Sanskrit in modern yoga classes is rampant, mostly because we English speakers tend to say the words as we would in English. But how important is precise pronunciation? Traditionally, it's extremely important in ritual performance. The underlying thought is that Sanskrit is a divine language, revealed to humans at the world's creation through the medium of inspired seers. As such, it embodies eternal truths that can only be expressed if the ritual words (or *mantras*) are accurately spoken or sung. Mispronunciation, we're warned, pollutes the offender's consciousness and, since each Sanskrit speaker is intimately bound through that language to both his religion and the universe, a flubbed word can have large-scale disastrous results.

In fact, during the ancient Vedic sacrifice, proper pronunciation of the ritual words was so essential that one of the priestly officiants, significantly named "the Brahman," was charged with monitoring the other priests. If there occurred any slip of the tongue during the recital, it was his job to immediately make amends, to ward off any retributive blowback from the heavens.

But this precision applies only to ritual Sanskrit. As Michael Coulson comments about everyday usage, most contemporary Sanskritists treat Sanskrit entirely as a written language, and when asked to pronounce a few words they usually don't bother to distinguish between closely related sounds. "How much trouble to take is thus a matter of personal choice," concludes Coulson, "*although the tendency nowadays is to pay more attention to such matters*" (italics mine).[20]

» *What are the most basic things I need to know about Sanskrit?*

So what does a non-Sanskritist need to know to have a halfway decent chance of approximating the correct pronunciation of Sanskrit? First there's what we might call the "one letter/syllable, one sound" rule. That is to say, unlike English letters, Sanskrit letters/syllables have one and only one way of being spoken. For example, at the start of an English word, the letter *c* can sound like a *k*, as in "cool," or an *s*, as in "cent." But the Sanskrit *ka* will always sound like "kuh," without exception. (I won't go through the pronunciation of all the letters/syllables here; it's easy enough to find a pronunciation guide online.)

It's also useful to know just where the accent falls in a word. But in order to understand how to accent a Sanskrit word, we first have to talk about the vowels, which play a determining role.

Sanskrit has thirteen vowels. Three of them (the *a, i,* and *u*) each have two forms, one "short" and one "long." The latter is marked with a macron, a short, horizontal line placed over the letter (*ā, ī, ū*) to distinguish it from its short companion. The long *ā*, both *i*'s, and both *u*'s are pronounced much like their English counterparts:

the short *a* = the first and last *a* in "America"
the long *ā* = the *a* in "father"
the short *i* = the *i* in "bit"
the long *ī* = *ee* in "see"
the short *u* = the *u* in "put"
the long *ū* = the *oo* in "coo"

PUNDIT/PANDIT

The English word "pundit" is the title given to recognized or self-appointed experts who pundi-ficate on a variety of subjects. In *nagari,* the word is spelled *pandit,* that is, with an *a* instead of a *u*. How did the *nagari a* become the English *u*? When an English speaker pronounces the word with the *a*-spelling, she would naturally tend to say, "pandit." But since the short *a* in Sanskrit is pronounced as *uh,* the earliest English speakers to visit India heard the word as "pun-dit," and so adjusted the spelling to suit their ear.

Here's some accent terminology you'll need to know. A syllable with a short vowel is called "light" (*laghu*); one with a long vowel or a diphthong is "heavy" (*guru*) (*e, ai, o, au*). A syllable is also heavy if its short vowel is followed by two or more consecutive consonants. Further, the next-to-last syllable in a word is called the penult, the one before that (the third syllable from the end) the ante-penult.

The accent in a Sanskrit word always falls on the heavy syllable, whether it's next to last (penult, second from the end), next to next-to-last (the ante-penult, third from the end), or—are you ready?—the next to next to next-to-last (the ante-ante-penult, the fourth from the end).

Here are a few examples:

1. heavy penult (*-yā-*): *abhyāsa*, "practice." Repeat after me: uh-BYAH-suh.
2. heavy penult (diphthong, *-she-*, the *-e-* pronounced as the *-ay* in "day"): *vishesha*, "difference." Repeat after me: vi-SHAY-shuh.
3. heavy penult (short vowel followed by two consecutive consonants, *-alp-*): *vikalpa*, "conceptualization." Repeat after me: vi-KUHL-puh.
4. light penult (*-va-*), heavy ante-penult (*īsh-*): *īshvara*, "lord, master." Repeat after me: EESH-vuh-ruh.
5. light penult (*-ya-*) and light ante-penult (*-par-*), accent on the ante-ante-penult (*vi-*): *viparyaya*, "misconception." Repeat after me: VI-puhr-yuh-yuh.

THE PALATAL *CA*

The Sanskrit syllable *ca* is no doubt in the Top Five of the most mispronounced syllables. Instead of the English sounding "see," *ca* sounds like the *ch* in "change," that is, *chuh*. For example: *cakra*, "wheel." Repeat after me: "chuck-ruh" (and not, as it's often mispronounced, *shock-ruh*).

Some translators, in order to help non-Sanskritists with their pronunciation, will transliterate *ca* as *cha*, so *cakra* is spelled *chakra* (or *citta* is spelled *chitta*, *candra* is spelled *chandra*, *brahmacarya* is spelled *brahmacharya*). But if *ca* is transliterated as *cha*, then *ca*'s aspirated companion, normally transliterated as *cha*, is forced to take another *h*. So for example *chaya*, "shadow," becomes *chhaya*. We won't run into this too often though, because words beginning with or containing *cha* are rare in yoga books (for an example, see *murccha* or "swooning" pranayama in HYP 2.44).

The retroflex consonants

Twenty-five of Sanskrit's thirty-three consonants are arranged in five groups of five consonants each. Professor Maurer notes that these are called "touched sounds"[21] because they involve one part of the mouth (usually the tongue) touching another. Each group of five consists of two pairs of consonants, one member of each pair being the aspirated form of its unaspirated companion (e.g., *k-kh, g-gh*), and a nasal (*ṅa, ña, ṇa, na,* and *ma*). The five groups are: the guttural, in which the tongue touches the back of the throat (Latin *guttur,* "throat"); palatal, in which the tongue touches the palate, the "roof of the mouth"; retroflex (more on this soon); dental, in which the tongue touches the teeth; and labial, in which the sound is made with the lips.

The names of the first, second, fourth, and fifth groups are fairly self-explanatory, but the name of the middle group, retroflex, needs some explanation. In transliteration, these consonants (*ṭa, ṭha, ḍa, ḍha, ṇa*) look almost exactly like the dentals, except for a little subscript dot that marks them as retroflex. To make these sounds, the curled-back tongue tip touches and then is sort of flicked off the roof of the mouth. These sounds are rather difficult to re-create in print, but Professor Maurer reassures us that an "acceptable approximation to these difficult sounds are the ordinary *t*'s and *d*'s of American English."[22]

HATHA

Most of us will recognize the retroflex *ṭha,* which is the second syllable of *haṭha. Haṭha* is almost always anglicized when pronounced, the first syllable *ha* made to rhyme with the English "Ma," the *ṭha* pronounced like the *th* in "the"; so it sounds something like "hah-the." But the "the" *th* sound doesn't exist in Sanskrit, and Sanskrit's short *a* sounds like *uh,* not *ah.* So repeat after me: huh-tuh, with the curled-back tongue flicked off the palate to pronounce the second syllable.

The semi-vowel *va*

Unlike all of the other consonants, the pronunciation of the semi-vowel *va* can be influenced by its position in a word. When it's the first syllable in a word, it's pronounced as the *v* in our "valve" or "villain." But when it follows a consonant in a sentence, in some parts of India, according to Professor Maurer, it's "pronounced approximately like a *w*," so *dvara,* "door," may be pronounced *dwara.*[23] For example: *svana,* "dog." Repeat after me: *swana* (shwa-nuh).

THE THREE SIBILANTS

Nagari has three sibilants or *s* sounds (*ś, ṣ, s*), the first is palatal (it's the only syllable marked with the accent acute), the second is retroflex (indicated by the subscript dot), and the third is dental. Although some Sanskrit primers make very subtle distinctions between the pronunciation of the first two syllables, for all intents and purposes they sound pretty much the same, like the *sh* in "shove." The dental *s* sounds just like the *s* in "so" (but *never* like the *z*-sounding *s* in "his"). We commonly see the palatal *ś* in words like *śava,* "corpse," and *śiva,* the name of the deity, the retroflex *ṣ* in *vrkṣa,* "tree," and *uṣtra,* "camel."

As we saw with *ca* transliterated as *cha,* the palatal and retroflex *s*'s are often transliterated as they sound, *sha,* or without their diacritical mark. So we might see *śava, shava,* or *sava,* and *uṣtra, ushtra,* or *ustra.* In the third spelling for both words, the undotted *-s-* is still pronounced *sh.*

SANSKRIT ODDITIES AND ENDS

Sanskrit enthusiasts heap praise on Sanskrit for its logical construction and ease of learning. There's no doubt some validity in these claims . . . only not for me. My experience over more than three years of informal but weekly study with a pair of tutors is that Sanskrit is mind-numbingly complex and absurdly quirky. Here are some of my favorite numbings and quirks.

THE SHORT *I*

The short *i* in *nagari* must certainly be one of the more unique letters in the entire history of the written word. That's because it's written *before* the consonant it's pronounced *after.* Let me put this in Roman letter terms with the word "pit." Were I to spell this word in *nagari,* the *i* would precede the *p* (*ipt*), though still be *pronounced* after it (in *nagari,* the *t* would have a special subscript mark negating its inherent *a*).

Apparently a very long time ago, both *i*'s were written as curls above their consonants, the short inclining to the left, the long to the right. At some point, to help distinguish one from the other, vertical lines were drawn down from the curls, so the line from the short curl preceded the consonant.

When writing in *nagari*, inexperienced Sanskritists (like yours truly) invariably fail to leave enough space in *front* of the consonant the short *i* is supposed to *follow*. This results in some frustrated erasing accompanied by an English commentary I'm quite sure has no equivalent Sanskrit translation.

THE SHORT *R*-VOWEL

You might wonder: what's an *r*-vowel? An *r* is a consonant, right? Well, there's an *r*-consonant in *nagari* (the only consonant that has its own name, *repha*, "passion"), but there's also an *r*-vowel (also called an *r*-colored vowel, a vocalic *r̥*, or liquid syllabic), marked by a subscript dot (the *r*-consonant and *r̥*-vowel are technically known as allophones, which means they're variants of the same basic speech sound or phoneme).

The story behind the vowel is long and complicated, and I'm not sure I understand it very well. Let's just say about this letter that it shows up in a few asana names. Probably the most familiar is *vr̥kṣa*, "tree," which might be spelled with an *i* after the *r̥* (*vrikṣa*) to help non-Sanskritists with their pronunciation, or (to give further help with the retroflex *ṣ*) *vriksha*. For most of us this is perfectly acceptable, though it seems not everyone agrees. The old-school American Sanskritist William Whitney decries it as "distorting and altogether objectionable."[24] According to Professor Maurer, the pronunciation of this vowel is much different today than it was long ago, and varies from one part of India to another. He says it's best just to pronounce it as we would an *r*-consonant. Michael Coulson believes it sounds more like the rolling *r* in the word "purdy," as in the Doris Day standard, "A Bushel and a Peck":

> . . . I love you a bushel and a peck
> You bet your purdy neck I do.

There's also a long *r̥*-vowel, marked with both a subscript dot and a macron, but to my knowledge it never occurs in any of the asana names.

THE Ḷ-VOWELS

The ḷ-vowel is another odd duck, or should I say rare bird. It appears in only one verb and its derivatives, *kḷp*, "to be well ordered or managed." Professor Maurer says that a "vocalic *ḷ* is heard in final *un*accented syllables of English words like *bottle*. . . . Nowadays, however, the pronunciation of *ḷ* is a strange amalgam of *ḷ* and *ṛ*, sounding much like *lru*."[25]

The ḷ-vowel technically has no long companion, though we might find it in some Sanskrit grammars, put there by Indian grammarians troubled by the uneven number of vowels and the gaping hole where the long ḷ-vowel, if there were one, would go.

THE *VISARGA*

The *visarga* ("send forth, emission") is written exactly like our colon (:), and transliterated as an *h* with a subscript dot *(ḥ)*. It usually comes at the tail end of a line of text or verse, following one of the simple vowels or a diphthong (*e, o, ai, au*). It's pronounced like an *h* with an echo of the previous simple vowel or *e* or *o*. So, for example, if the previous vowel is a short *a*, the *visarga* sounds like ah[a] (ah-ha), if it's a short *u* it sounds like uh[u] (uh-huh). The *ai* and *au* are a bit different, in that only the second of the two transliterated letters (*i* and *u*) is pronounced; for example: aiḥ = aih[i] (eye-high).

We have a *visarga* at the end of one of the most famous verses in all of yoga, *Yoga Sutra* 1.2: *yogaś citta vṛtti nirodhaḥ* (yo-gush chit-tuh vrit-tee ni-row-duh-huh), "yoga is the restriction of the fluctuations of consciousness."

SANDHI ("JUNCTION")

Another Sanskrit oddity is called "junction" or "connection" (*sandhi*), what the dictionary defines as a "euphonic coalition." This means that when one word follows another in a sentence, the last letter/syllable of the first word affects and is affected by the first letter/syllable of the second (this is called external *sandhi*; there's also an internal *sandhya* affecting letters within a word, which we'll pass on). This ensures that the sounds of the words will combine in a pleasing way.

We see *sandhi* in the names of the asanas all the time. Take the sitting twist called *matsyendra* (I've left off the *asana*). It's composed of two smaller words, *matsya* ("fish") and *indra* (typically interpreted "lord"). As you can see, when the final *a* of *matsya* reacts with the initial *i* of *indra,* by the rules of *sandhi* the two letters blend to an *e.* Here are three common *sandhis* you'll find in asanas:

> final short *a* + initial short *a* = a long *ā.* This is probably the most common *sandhi.* Example: *trikona* + *asana* = *trikonāsana.* Here the initial *a* of *asana* blends with the final *a* of the posture's main name, *trikona* ("triangle").
> final *a* + initial *e* = *ai.* Example: *mukha eka pada* = *mukhaikapada*
> final *a* + initial *u* = *o.* Example: *pashcima* + *uttana* = *pashcimottana*

Maybe the *sandhi* is not so odd after all, since we do have something similar in spoken English. For example, if I say the sentence, " I want to go," unless I enunciate each word carefully, it'll probably come out sounding something like, "I wanna go." The blending of "want" and "to" might be considered a "euphonic coalition." The difference in Sanskrit is that, unlike English, the blending of letters and words is reflected in the writing. One major result of *sandhi,* by the way, is that Sanskrit sentences or verses can roll merrily along for line after line withoutanyinterveningspaces. This can, says Professor Maurer, cause "considerable difficulty for the beginner in Sanskrit" (no kidding) who can't as yet "readily discern the word junctures" that will presumably, one hopes, be "immediately apparent at a later stage." Why is Sanskrit written this way? In the old days, it was possibly to "conserve writing material"—after all, spaces take up, um, space—but most of all, Professor Maurer continues, because *nagari* is actually easier to write when using the special vowel signs that follow consonants and by joining consonants together at word junctures.[26] Nowadays in Sanskrit books in which the *nagari* is transliterated into the Roman alphabet, considerate editors will often take pity on novices and hyphenate-the-sentences-or-verses-to-make-them-more-easily-readable.

Sandhi isn't the only joining going on in Sanskrit; there's also something called *samyoga,* "yoked together." Whenever one consonant immediately follows another (with no intervening vowel), the two are combined or "yoked." Sometimes it's easy enough to tell (or guess) which two letters are being yoked in this way: they'll more or less retain their unyoked shape. Other times though, the yoking creates a completely new character. For example, when the syllables (j) and (n) combine, as in the word *jnana,* "wisdom," the character (*ñ*) is formed.

This means that in addition to the forty-eight basic characters of the *nagari* alpha-syllabary, we also have to learn at least sixty of the more common "conjunct" consonants, though an informal count of "consonant clusters" in one Sanskrit primer yielded over 280 (!) different yoked consonants.

» *Could you go over the Peacock misprint in* Light on Yoga*?*

Pīncha means the chin or a feather.

B. K. S. IYENGAR, *Light on Yoga*, p. 170

Very early in my yoga career, I was taught that the Sanskrit name of what we informally called the forearm or elbow balance was *pincha mayurasana,* literally the "peacock feather pose." The name, which appeared in Mr. Iyengar's famous yoga manual, *Light on Yoga*, was no doubt suggested by the inverted practitioner's raised legs reaching up out of the torso, which resembles, if we use our imagination, the fanned tail of the peacock.

I had no reason to question this name, since it was backed by the unquestioned (and unquestionable) authority of Mr. Iyengar, and for many years I dutifully repeated this tidbit of information, that *pincha* meant "feather," to my students, always adding for good measure that *pincha* "also means chin." Not long ago, while helping a friend with some writing, out of curiosity I decided to check on *pincha* in an online Sanskrit-English dictionary. Much to my surprise, when I searched with the accepted spelling of the word, the response I got was "No entries found." I assumed I'd misspelled the word, so I tried again, and again received the same response. Now quite confused but at the same time intrigued, I opened one of those old-fashioned paper dictionaries and flipped around in the general vicinity of *pī-*.

The reason for the missing *pincha* soon became evident: there's no such word, at least not spelled exactly in that way. The *n* in *pīncha* is classified as a "dental" consonant (with the tongue touching the teeth), but it should rather be a "palatal" *n*, the only consonant crowned with a tilde (~), and pronounced like the *n* in punch. The problem with *this* word, in turn, is that it doesn't mean "feather," it means "wing." I then went to an English-Sanskrit dictionary and looked up the word "feather," the Sanskrit equivalent of which is *piccha* (which also can mean "wing, tail, crest"). And so we have three choices when deciding what to call his pose. We can continue to call it by its incorrect though widely accepted name, and not rock the boat. Or else we can rock the boat, probably in the face of widespread protest, and rename the pose either *piñcha* or *piccha mayurasana,* with the understanding that if we choose that first alternative, the pose will then be translated literally as "peacock wing pose."

I haven't been able to ascertain how or why *piñcha/piccha* became *pīncha.* Quite possibly it's a misprint. Every author knows that such minor slip-ups can occur in even the most carefully copyedited book. The problem with this explanation is that *pīncha* not only doesn't mean "feather," it doesn't mean "chin" either. The English-Sanskrit dictionary provides several possibilities for "chin," like *chubuka, cibi, hanu,* and *joda,* none of which are even close to being spelled like *pīncha.*

» Is it true the modern brand name Viagra is derived from the Sanskrit word vyaghra, "tiger"?

Viagra is a drug used to treat pulmonary arterial hypertension and, well, what's formally known as male "erectile dysfunction." It's been suggested by more than one person that the name derives from the Sanskrit word for "tiger," *vyaghra.* If we Google "vyaghra viagra," we're presented with over eleven thousand responses, most of them websites selling the little blue, diamond-shaped pill. But a good number also address this question, which has actually generated no small amount of controversy. The answers fall naturally into three groups: no, it doesn't; maybe yes, maybe no; and yes, it does.

The "no" group is convinced the similarity between the two words is a cosmic coincidence, plain and simple. Viagra to them is nothing more than a trade name, concocted like all such names to simplify the drug's generic name (which, incidentally, is sildenafil citrate, a name that certainly cries out for simplification), or to indicate something about the condition it treats.

The "maybe" group, as the name implies, straddles the Viagra-*vyaghra* fence. Like agnostics everywhere, they're willing to be swayed in either direction by conclusive evidence. Some allow that Viagra has a suspiciously close affinity with the Sanskrit word; but then again, they add, it also rhymes with "Niagara," as in Niagara Falls, a popular honeymoon destination where presumably the pill is in high demand. Couldn't that be the inspiration for the name?

The "yes" group views the no's and maybe's with the same attitude that we may view someone who believes the earth is flat. My gosh, they say, just *look* at the two words: how can you call that a coincidence, and what is there to doubt?

There was one response to this question that I especially enjoyed, and I suppose it belongs with the "no" group. The person, obviously a Sanskritist of some experience, pointed out that *vyaghra*, with its long *a* and aspirated *g*, sounds nothing like its supposed English cousin.

Incidentally, is there a Tiger Pose (*vyaghrasana*)? There is indeed. In fact I found at least three different versions, two of which are described and illustrated in Mr. Iyengar's *Light on Yoga* under different names. One is called Lion Pose II (*simhasana* II, LoY 50), in which the practitioner, from Lotus, leans forward onto the inner knees and hands, with elbows straight, and performs the familiar cross-eyed, tongue-protruding roar of Lion Pose I. The other goes by the name of Bhairava's Pose (*bhairavasana*, LoY 375). It's performed lying face up with one leg wrapped around the back of the neck. The third variation is found in yoga teacher Dharma Mitra's little black book, *Asanas: 608 Yoga Poses* (plate 363), where it appears as Tiger Pose (*vyaghrasana*). Mitra performs it on hands and knees, first drawing a bent knee up into his chest as he rounds his back, then stretching that same leg straight out behind his torso as he arches his back (there are several variations shown as well).

Nagari has no punctuation except a single vertical bar (|), called a "stick" (*daṇḍa*), that marks the end of a half-verse or sentence, and a double stick (||), the end of a full verse or paragraph ||

3

SACRED
KNOWLEDGE
What Is the Veda?

Who saw the newborn one, the one with bones who was
brought forth by the boneless one? Where was the breath
and blood and soul of the earth? Who can go to ask this
from someone who knows? An ignorant fool, I ask in my
mind about the hidden footprints of the gods.

Questions (but no answers) from the *Rig Veda*, 1.164.4–5

THE UPANISHADS ARE A collection of texts that chronologically
come at the tail end of an even larger collection of texts known as the
Veda. This word derives from the root *vid*, "to know," so Veda literally
means "knowledge" or, to be more precise, sacred knowledge (*vid* is at the
root of English words like "vision," "view," "evident," "survey").

VEDA

Similar to the word *sutra* (see Chapter 4), "Veda" has a dual application. It can refer to either the entire collection of books (i.e., the Veda)
or just one of the four earliest texts in the collection, the *Rig Veda,
Sama Veda, Yajur Veda,* and *Atharva Veda* (more on each of these
coming up).

The foundation of the entire Vedic edifice is a book titled the *Rig Veda,* the "knowledge of Praise." (How the Sanskrit word for praise, *rc,* becomes *rig* is a long story involving the effect certain Sanskrit words have on those around them; suffice it to say that when *rc* is followed by the *v* of Veda, it turns into *rg,* which for the sake of non-Sanskritists and their reading pleasure, I'm spelling *rig.*) Two more books are closely related to the *Rig Veda,* since it's the source of most of their material. These books are the "knowledge of Sacrifice" (*Yajur Veda*) and the "knowledge of chants" (*Sama Veda*).

A fourth book is associated with these three, though it has by no means, even after a very long time, achieved total acceptance by Vedic scholars. This is the *Atharva Veda,* named after the priest Atharvan, said to be the first priest to worship fire. The three other Vedas might be compared to respectable family members, while the *Atharva Veda,* with its spells and charms, is the black sheep of the family. Its material is divided into two groups. One consists of malevolent (*abhicara*) spells, used to unhinge enemies with some horrible illness or impossibly bad luck (you might already have someone in mind you'd like to target). The other describes remedial (*bheshajani*) charms to treat various virulent diseases, personified—maybe a better word is demonified—as flesh-eating ogres (*pishacha*) and devils (*rakshasa*). Here's one such charm, rebuking the dreaded fever demon, Takman:

> And thou thyself who makest all men yellow, consuming them with burning heat. . . . Thou, Fever! Then be weak and ineffective. Pass hence into the realms below or vanish.

There are also charms for successful childbirth (especially for sons); for love affairs and the revival of virility (the Vedic equivalent of Viagra); for a long life, up to a "hundred autumns"; to expiate sins and create family harmony; to bring farmers rain, to shield shepherds and their herds from wild animals, and to protect merchants from robbers. There are even charms to bring good luck to gamblers and, as Sanskritist Maurice Bloomfield (1855–1928) amusingly writes, "charms calculated to promote the interests of the Brahmins, especially to secure for them the abundant baksheesh [what we nowadays call a "tip," likely for ritual services rendered] for which they clamor with most refreshing directness." But

Professor Bloomfield doesn't dismiss the *Atharva Veda* completely, acknowledging it as having "unrivaled importance for the history of superstition, of folk-lore, and popular practices."[1]

The *Rig Veda* consists of ten chapters or "circles" (*mandalas*) with just over a thousand *suktas* ("well said, eloquent"), totaling almost eleven thousand verses. My edition, translated in the late nineteenth century by British Sanskritist Ralph Griffith (available online),[2] runs to just over 650 pages of eye-squinting type (this includes also a running commentary). The sheer length of the text is remarkable, which makes it then even more remarkable that originally, before writing developed in India in perhaps the third or fourth century B.C.E., the entire text was memorized by Vedic priests and passed along orally for countless generations.

SUKTAS AND HYMNS

The *Rig Veda*'s *suktas* are often called hymns, but that's a bit misleading, at least to us Westerners. In our services a hymn is usually sung communally, but the suktas of the *Rig Veda* are chanted exclusively by the presiding priests.

Have you ever played a game called Rumors (or sometimes Telephone)? You need a pretty good crowd of people to make it work best. One person starts a "rumor," which she whispers into her neighbor's ear. Her neighbor then whispers what he's heard (or thinks he's heard) into his neighbor's ear, and so on around the room. Finally, the last person to hear the rumor reports it to the gathering. If you've ever participated in this game you know what the typical outcome is—the end rumor has little or no relationship to the beginning rumor; each person in the group has taken what he or she has heard and interpreted (or embellished it) in his or her own way. The game itself is a lesson in how easy it is to change or confuse an oral tale. Now consider that the *Rig Veda* was passed on orally across hundreds of years, with hardly any distortion whatsoever!

All of the Vedas are very old, though exactly how old is a matter of heated dispute. Western scholars tend to date the *Rig Veda* at somewhere between 3,200 and 3,500 years old. Indian traditionalists and their Western sympathizers, as we have seen, firmly believe these dates are grossly underestimated; some of these folks take the earliest suktas of the *Rig Veda* back six thousand years. The hard-core traditionalists maintain that dating the *Rig Veda* is an enormous waste of time, because the contents of the book are eternal, recited by the creator deity, Brahma, to selected seers (*rishis*) at the beginning of each world cycle. It's for this reason that the Veda is called *shruti*, "what is heard," its wisdom (much like the holy books of Western religions) believed to be infallible. As such, it occupies a special niche in Hindu spiritual literature, forever separate from the texts produced by fallible human authors, called *smriti*, "what is remembered."

LINEAR VS. CYCLICAL TIME

Our Western Judeo-Christian conception of time is linear. According to this view, the world is created at Point A, runs through its life cycle, and then (so it's predicted), at some distant Point B in the future, there's a day of reckoning when all souls are called to judgment and sent to their final reward, presumably for all eternity.

By contrast, Indian time is cyclical. If we compare Western time to a freight train chugging one way down a track, then time in India is a carousel, and the world goes "round and round and round" like Joni Mitchell's "circle game." Every creation is followed eventually by a dissolution, every dissolution by a new creation. Incidentally, the end of a world cycle is often described as its destruction, but that's not exactly accurate; rather, at the end of its appointed cycle, the world is resolved back into the primal matrix (*pradhana*, "primary germ, the original source of the material world"), where it's recycled to be used for the next round. This is technically called a *pralaya*, "dissolution, reabsorption."

The question of the Veda's age isn't the only controversy that pits Western scholars against Indian traditionalists. The former group tends to dismiss the Rig as nothing much more than a collection of nature poetry, much of it second-rate at that, though they do discern here and there the stirring of some "higher" spiritual awareness. Indian traditionalists are absolutely incensed by this estimation, which to them once more displays

Western scholars' obtuseness when it comes to the Indian spirit. The suktas, writes Judith Tyberg (who speaks for her guru, Sri Aurobindo and Western scholar-teacher David Frawley), are addressed to the "Devas or Gods of the Elements and the Phenomena of Nature, but [are] also symbolic of aspiring prayers to the subtler and higher in man."[3] Traditionalists firmly believe that the songs were purposely written to seem like primitive poetry, to conceal the revelatory wisdom from individuals who, for one reason or another, are unqualified to receive their teachings.

This "hidden message" is what the revered Indian sage Sri Aurobindo (1872–1950) calls the "secret of the Veda" (and the title of one of his books, first published in installments in the monthly review *Arya* between 1914 and 1920). Aurobindo writes that the Veda's suktas, condemned by Western scholars as "obscure and barbarous compositions," have been the "source not only of some of the world's richest and profoundest religions, but some of its subtlest metaphysical philosophies."[4]

I certainly don't have the training to make a decision about who is right and wrong here, but we have to admit, when we read something like the following, it's hard to deny that the ancient seers and poets didn't have at least an inkling of the divine.

> There was neither non-existence nor existence then; there was neither the realm of space nor the sky which is beyond. What stirred? Where? In whose protection? Was there water, bottomlessly deep? . . . Who really knows? Who will here proclaim it? Whence was it produced? . . . Whence this creation has arisen—perhaps it formed itself, or perhaps it did not—the one who looks down on it, in the highest heaven, only he knows—or perhaps he does not know.
>
> *Rig Veda* 10.129 (translation by Wendy Doniger)

The foregoing is only a very shallow scratch on the surface of the subject of the Veda. We didn't go into the poets who wrote the Rig's suktas, how the suktas were arranged, how the four "collections" (*samhita*) were each used during rituals and sacrifices, or what the sacrifices themselves were intended to achieve.

What's important for us to know in regard to yoga is the direction the Vedic rituals took over time, and the resulting consequences. Initially the rituals were quite simple, but gradually became more and more complex—the number of priests at one sacrifice, for example, grew from four to sixteen—and so, not surprisingly, more and more expensive, until only the wealthiest of the wealthy could afford to sponsor one (it would seem that making lots of money off spiritual services isn't just a modern innovation). The priests then became even more secretive with and protective of the samhitas, now that they not only embodied the word of god but were the source of a highly lucrative income. It's said that even after writing developed in India in the third or fourth century B.C.E., the priests refused to write down the suktas, fearing that a physical book would be much easier to acquire than the contents of one of their caste's memory banks.

So as centuries passed and the rituals became more convoluted, their original meaning grew less clear or was lost altogether. This resulted in a burgeoning commentarial literature, the purpose of which was to help each succeeding generation of priests understand what they were up to and why. These commentaries, each appended to one of the four samhitas, are known as the Brahmanas.

» What are the Brahmanas?

The Brahmanas are usually said to be so named because they were written by and for Brahmin priests. The oldest prose works written in any Indo-European language, they've been called the Hindu Talmud. They aren't, however, considered great literature, at least by Western scholars. Professor Winternitz allows that, for the student of religion, they are "indispensable to the understanding of the whole of later religious and philosophical literature of the Indians." He concludes, though, that as just reading they are "unpalatable,"[5] a judgment that, compared with some of the others made by fellow scholars, is rather mild. There are about a dozen Brahmanas, each one appended to one of the samhitas, and each with two parts: a "rule" (*vidhi*) part, which details rules or regulations for the proper conduct of the complex ceremonies or sacrifices; and an expository (*artha vada*) part, a what-not of explanations for the origins of the rituals and the legends connected with them.

» *What are the "Forest Books"* (Aranyaka*)?*

Not everyone in the Brahmin community was engaged in shoring up the ritual and maybe even cashing in. There were Brahmins who weren't priests (along with some who were) who'd grown dissatisfied with the direction the Vedic rituals had taken. Joined by educated members of the nobility (which included the warrior class), along with a variety of world renouncers (including Buddhists) and doctrinal skeptics, they began to ask themselves, in Professor Winternitz's words, the "highest questions"[6]; that is, they began the search, which continues today, for the answer to the only question, in the end, that matters: Who am I?

The result was another level of appendices, these attached to the Brahmanas, known as the "Forest Books" (*Aranyaka*). But unlike those mostly dry, unreadable commentaries (again, according to Western scholars), this new level "comprised everything which was of a secret, uncanny character," no longer interested in rules and explanations for the ritual, but the "mysticism and symbolism of the sacrifice."[7] The Forest Books, in other words, began the move (completed in the Upanishads) to internalize the outward physical ritual and all of its paraphernalia, and transformed it "from the brooding on the wonder of the outside world to the meditation on the significance of the self."[8]

There's some disagreement about the meaning of the collective name of these books. Most scholars believe they are so named because they were written by forest-dwelling hermits and ascetics, living outside the pale not only of Vedic ritualism but Vedic culture in general. Others, though, like Professor Winternitz, maintain that, because of their anti-ritualistic stance, which surely must have antagonized the Brahmin priests, and their dangerous teachings, they could only be safely "taught and learned in the forest," away from the prying ears in the villages.[9]

> *I get mixed messages about yoga and the* Rig Veda.
> *Some scholars say it's taught there, other say it's not.*
> *What do you think? Is there any yoga teaching to be*
> *found in the Rig?*

Though the evidence is rather slim, both Georg Feuerstein and scholar-teacher David Frawley believe that, yes, there's evidence of yoga in the *Rig Veda*. Feuerstein bases his case for Rig Vedic Yoga on a number of suktas that hint at what seem suspiciously like yogic activities. For example, he detects a potential forerunner of later generations of yogis in the wandering ascetic celebrated in the "Hymn of the Long-haired One":

> The long-haired one is said to gaze full on heaven, the long-haired one is said to be that light.
> The wind-girt sages have donned the yellow robe of dust; along the wind's course they glide when the gods have penetrated them.
>
> *Rig Veda* 10.136 (translation by Jeanine Miller)

Of course any "yoga" that was practiced back in Vedic times, maybe three thousand years ago or more, doubtless had little or nothing in common with what passes for "yoga" today. But it's entirely possible that many of our yoga exercises were born in the rituals of the Vedic sages and priests. Certainly the sacrifice demanded alertness and precision of speech, breath, and movement, and a mind "harnessed" intently on the god being solicited. Indeed, in the *Chandogya Upanishad* (1.10.8), it's said that if a priest sings a hymn "without knowing the divinity" connected with it, his "head will fall off"—no doubt a powerful incentive to concentrate on the matter at hand.

There are other possible Vedic sources of later yogic practices. Since the priest reciting the suktas needed to pronounce them precisely to gain the gods' favor, it's very likely that the priest had to consciously control his breath. Dr. Feuerstein ventures that such breath control may have induced a profound shift in his awareness, which foreshadowed later yoga schools' work with monitored breathing or pranayama.

Professor Winternitz mentions that, when learning the verses, the student-priest emphasized various notes "by means of movements of the hands and fingers."[10] Similar gestures were also used to count the recitation of Vedic vocal tones. Could it be that these ritual hand movements are the precursors of the hand seals (*hasta mudras*, see Chapter 5) or symbolic gestures we make in our practice?

» *What are the Upanishads?*

> Give not that which is holy unto the dogs, neither cast ye your pearls before swine, lest they trample them under their feet, and turn again and rend you.
>
> MATTHEW 7:6

Despite the porous boundaries between the Aranyakas and the Upanishads, these latter books are considered the "end" (*anta*) of the Veda in two senses. Physically (and chronologically) they're the "last chapter" of the Veda, and philosophically they're the goal or culmination of the Vedic teaching. In these two senses, the teaching contained in the Upanishads is known as the "end of the Veda," or Vedanta.

Since they weren't written for a popular audience, the Upanishads aren't the easiest read in the world. Many of the books are compilations of shorter teachings by different teachers, and they were probably tinkered with and maybe modified by several editors, sometimes of divergent philosophical or spiritual agendas. As a result, the language can be choppy and the teaching unsystematic, occasionally even contradictory.

Then, too, to folks like us, the language of the Upanishads can be obscure or seemingly nonsensical. While the confusion caused by hit-and-miss editing was unintentional, language laden with analogies, doublespeak, symbols, metaphors and similes, and parables wasn't. Called "twilight speech" (*sandhya bhasha*), such language is designed to further veil and protect the teaching; even if one of us outsiders somehow manages to hear a bit of it, without the key to the language's code, it would all be Greek—or better yet, Sanskrit—to us.

But twilight language not only *con*ceals, it also *re*veals ... but again only if you have the key. It first obliges the student to give his undivided attention to what is being said, which induces a kind of meditative state. Then it pushes the student to think, as we say, "outside the box," to dismantle habitual modes of consciousness and open himself to new possibilities, while it allows the author of the text to approximate in words what is essentially ineffable.

The length of each Upanishad varies widely. The *Isha Upanishad* could fit in your palm, covering a little more than two pages in one of my translations, while the *Brihad Aranyaka Upanishad* meanders along (in one modern edition for eighty-seven pages). Like most of the books of early India, the names of the authors (or at least the contributors) are forever lost (if they were ever known), though key teachings commemorate famous teachers like Yajnavalkya, Svetaketu, and Shandilya.

» *What does the word "Upanishad" mean?*

Upanishad (*upa* = near; *ni* = down; *sat* = to sit) [means] literally sitting down near the Guru to receive spiritual instruction.

B. K. S. IYENGAR, *Light on the Yoga
Sutras of Patanjali* (1993), p. 327

The word *upanishad* is composed of the verbal root *sat* ("to sit") prefixed with *upa* and *ni,* and means "to sit down close to (one's teacher)."

GEORG FEUERSTEIN, *The Shambhala
Encyclopedia of Yoga* (2011), p. 315

. . . it is meaningless to say . . . that the word *Upanishad* denotes knowledge acquired "by sitting at the feet of a teacher"; this title, if such were the meaning, would then apply without distinction to all parts of the Veda; moreover, it is an interpretation which has never been suggested or admitted by any competent Hindu. In reality, the name of the Upanishads denotes that they are ordained to destroy ignorance by providing the means to supreme Knowledge.

RENE GUENON, *Man and His Becoming* (1981), p. 23

The Sanskrit word *upanishad* consists of three smaller words, *upa, ni,* and *shad.* The first two are prefixes meaning, respectively, "toward, near to, by the side of," and "down." For our purposes, *shad* can mean "to sit" (*shad* is cognate with our English word, "sit"), "to place down," or "to destroy." By far and away the most popular interpretation of *upanishad* is "to sit down near." This is said to hark back to the time, long ago, when the spiritual teacher delivered his message to the initiated student orally, the two sitting face-to-face in isolation.

It may seem shocking to us, accustomed as we are to the impartial dissemination of yoga knowledge to all and sundry, but once upon a time, such knowledge wasn't available to just anybody. The teachings were thought to be imbued with magical power, and if they fell into the wrong hands, so to speak, they could have one of two dire consequences: they could blow up in the face of a poorly or untrained individual, or be used by an unscrupulous character against others. Denied then to the general public and reserved only for mature students trusted not to let the cat out of the bag, the word *upanishad* also acquired the symbolic meaning of *rahasya*, "secret, concealed."

Other interpretations have been championed for the word *upanishad*. Indian authorities, such as Shankara (ca. 788–822 C.E.), the great exponent of Advaita (nondual) Vedanta (see Chapter 4 on Vedanta), proposed it meant to set at rest (or destroy) self-ignorance by "revealing the knowledge of the supreme spirit." This view has been rejected by the scholarly crowd; Sanskritist and Indologist Arthur Keith, for example, maintains this interpretation defies the "laws of etymology,"[11] though he doesn't say why.

There are a handful of reputable scholars, though, who make a strong case for an interpretation of *upanishad* entirely different from "to sit down near." I first ran across this position in a 2002 PhD thesis, "History, Text, and Context of the Yoga Upanishads," by Jeffrey Ruff.[12] He writes: "The word *upanishad* is a technical term in early Indian esotericism. The primary meaning is . . . 'connection,' 'homology,' or 'equivalence.'" Then he continues:

From the Sanskrit roots upa + ni + sad, the terms were formerly misunderstood to mean "to sit close beside". . . . This characterization has been so widely disseminated since . . . [the] 1890s . . . that one will find it in almost every introduction to the texts, both

Western and Indian. It is a misleading though largely harmless interpretation.[13]

It certainly was a relief to me to know that the misinformation I'd been passing on to trusting students for the past twenty-eight years was "largely harmless," and that none of my students are likely to suffer irreparable upanishadic trauma. I thought it wise, however, to get a second opinion in this matter, so I decided to check with a more established authority. Several times in his thesis, Ruff cites Patrick Olivelle, a Humanities professor at the University of Texas and a Sanskritist with a resume that includes two translations of and commentaries on various Upanishads. In one of his translations he writes that the older view "that the term derives from 'sitting near' a teacher and refers to a group of disciples at the feet of a teacher imbibing esoteric knowledge is clearly untenable."[14]

Now with all due respect to Professor Olivelle, I wouldn't go so far as to claim that the "sit down near" interpretation is "clearly untenable," since it's readily accepted by many highly qualified Sanskritists, Indiaphiles, and yoga teachers. I decided to get a third opinion and turned to another expert cited by Ruff, Louis Renou, a French Indologist. In his 1953 work, *Religions of Ancient India*, Renou succinctly states that the "word *upanishad* . . . means only 'equivalence,'"[15] while eight years later in *Hinduism*, a book he edited, he changes the meaning of the word to "approaches."[16]

What are Ruff, Olivelle, and Renou getting at here? "To sit down near" refers to a literal event, where the student goes to get a lesson from the teacher. What Ruff et al. are saying is that *upanishad* should be instead interpreted figuratively, in the sense of "putting two things down near each other" for the purpose of making a statement by comparing one to the other.

So where did this mistake come from? Olivelle lays it at the feet of a German Indologist, Paul Deussen (1845–1919), who, writing in 1898 in *The Philosophy of the Upanishads*, initiated the whole supposed mix-up by proclaiming in his most authoritative Teutonic voice:

> For *upanishad,* derived as a substantive from the root *sad,* can only denote a "sitting"; and as the preposition *upa* (near by) indicates . . . a "confidential secret sitting."[17]

Now we can understand how the mistake got traction. Deussen was a respected Sanskritist and Orientalist, so his words carried some weight and people would tend to believe him without question. But Renou's book, *Religions of Ancient India*, with the above revised definition of *upanishad*, first came out in 1953, more than sixty years ago. If he was such a preeminent Indologist, why did his contradiction of "sit down near by" fail to take root and supplant Deussen's translation?

» *How many Upanishads are there?*

Tradition counts 108, though in fact scholars cite numbers from 120 to over 200. One-hundred-eight is a sacred number that crops up continually in the yoga tradition (see Chapter 5), though what it actually signifies is up in the air. Dr. Feuerstein believes that 108 is linked with the number eighteen, which in Hindu symbolism represents wholeness or completeness (as in the eighteen chapters of the great Indian epic poem, the *Mahabharata,* and the eighteen chapters of the *Bhagavad Gita*). The word *shri,* an honorific prefix meaning "sacred, holy," is sometimes written 108 times before the name of a revered teacher.

In the end it doesn't really matter how many Upanishads there are, since only ten to thirteen are typically considered principal (*mukhya*). They're deemed so because they were commented on by the aforementioned sage-philosopher Shankara. Once more the experts disagree, in this case about which of the Upanishads should be labeled "principal," but we can safely list the following thirteen (in roughly chronological order) without ruffling too many scholarly feathers:

Brhad Aranyaka Upanishad ("Great Forest")
Chandogya Upanishad, a word derived by combining *chandas,* "hymn" (but also "desire, longing for"), and *ga,* "singing"; in plain English, this title indicates that the book's teaching follows the *chandoga,* the "metrical singer" of the *Sama Veda.*
Taittiriya Upanishad (from *tittiri,* "partridge") of the *Black Yajur Veda*
Kaushitaki Upanishad, named after a Brahmin family in which teaching was handed down

Aitareya Upanishad, named after a sage

Kena Upanishad, named after the first word of the book, *kena,* "by whom?"

Katha Upanishad, named after a sage, one of the disciples of Vaisampayana and, perhaps, one of the partridges of the *Black Yajur Veda* (see accompanying Yoga Story)

Shvetashvatara, a word derived by combining *shveta,* "white," and *ashva,* "horse"; put these together and you get "White Horse." Dr. Feuerstein comments that this title applies to someone whose senses, which are said to resemble wild horses, are purified and controlled. Other scholars maintain that it's the name of a teacher, literally the "man with a white mule."

Isha, named after the first word of the book, *isha,* "by the Lord"

Mundaka Upanishad (from *munda,* "shaved, bald"). There are some interesting differences of opinion about this title. The simplest explanation, from Professor Winternitz, is that the text is meant only for ascetics with shaved heads (rather than clutter this short entry with footnotes, I'll include all sources under one note at the end). The shaved head, says Valerie Roebuck, is a visible sign that the person has renounced the world (as it is in many religions around the world). S. Radhakrishnan interprets the bald pate symbolically: it shows the ascetic has "shaved off" or liberated himself from "error and ignorance."

A rather controversial interpretation of the shaved head involves something called the "head vow" (*shirovratam*). In order to gain access to the Mundaka text, writes Benjamin Walker (and seconded by V. M. Bedekar and G. B. Palsule), the ascetic is required to hold a basin with hot coals or embers over his shaved head. This is supposed to symbolize the "heat" of knowledge that will descend on him from the teaching. Patrick Olivelle sums it up neatly, saying that while all of this is plausible, none of it is certain.[18]

Prashna, literally "question, demand, interrogation," named for the six questions asked of the sage Pippalada by six learned Brahmins, regarding creation, the "life breath" (*prana*), how the life breath travels into and through the body, dreaming and dreamless sleep, the value of meditating on the syllable OM, and the sixteen "parts" of a human (which are life breath, faith, space, wind, light, water, earth, senses, mind, food, strength, austerity, mantra, sacrifice, worlds, and name, that is, individuals)

Maitrayaniya (from *maitri*, "friendliness, benevolence")

Mandukya (from *manduka*, "frog"), the name of a sage. Alternatively, one scholar suggests this Upanishad is so named because it belonged to a group of people whose totem animal was a frog, and that the god Varuna, who is associated with this book, once took the form of a frog.

YOGA STORY

The Partridge and the Horse: Two Versions of the *Yajur Veda*

The Yajur (*yajus*, "sacrificial formula") exists in two versions called the *Black (krishna) Yajur Veda* (also known as the *Taittiriya Samhita*) and the *White (shukla) Yajur Veda* (*Vajasaneyi Samhita*). While the Black and White are treated as separate books, there really isn't much difference in content between them. According to one scholar, the Black has some theological discussions of the sacrifices that the White doesn't.

There's a legend recounting how the *Yajur Veda* was split. Once upon a time there was a *Yajur* priest by the name of Vaisampayana, the son of Vyasa, the legendary "author" not only of the *Rig Veda* but of the great epic poem, the *Mahabharata*, the longest poem in the world. Vaisampayana had committed a grave offense, accidentally causing the death of his sister's child, and asked his twenty-seven disciples to help him with his penance. One disciple, Yajnavalkya, insisted that he expiate his teacher's sin by himself. Vaisampayana, miffed at this impertinence, cursed Yajnavalkya, who then immediately, um, *disgorged* all the Yajur material he'd learned in, uh, *tangible* form.

When Vaisampayana ordered the other disciples to clean up the mess, they transformed themselves into partridges (*tittiri*) and swallowed what Yajnavalkya had regurgitated. The resulting book was called the *Black Yajur Veda*, apparently because it was "soiled" or stained with blood, or the *Taittiriya Samhita*, literally the "collection of the partridges." Yajnavalkya then prayed to the Sun, who appeared to Yajnavalkya in the shape of a horse (*vajin*), and imparted a new and improved version of the Yajur. This book was called the *White Yajur Veda* or the *Vajasaneyi Samhita*, literally the "collection of the horse."

UPANISHADIC CATEGORIES

The presumed 108 Upanishads are sometimes divided into seven categories. Different sources number the texts in each category slightly differently. Along with the principal Upanishads, the other six categories are: Vedantic, Samnyasa ("renunciation"), Shakta (relating to the goddess Devi), Vaishnava (relating to Vishnu), Shaiva (relating to Shiva), and Yoga. This last category, usually numbering twenty-one texts, is of special interest to yoga students.

As you might expect, considering their evolution, the Upanishads are a virtual crazy quilt of all kinds of information, from the most sublime to the most mundane. You'll find (in no particular order): teachings on ritual, sacrifice, mantras (especially OM), and a few charms; debates and dialogues between teacher and student, father and son, even husband and wife (see below); creation and end-of-world accounts; teaching stories, legends, and parables; aphorisms and precepts; esoteric anatomy (like the energetic channels, the *nadis*, of the subtle body, which play a central role in Hatha Yoga), the correspondences between the microcosm (the human body) and the macrocosm (the world), and the vital breath (*prana*); highly imaginative etymologies; speculation on the nature or "warp" of world, of the Self (*atman*), and of ultimate reality (*brahman*); death, life-after-death, and transmigration; sleep, dream, and waking states; teacher lineages; the theory of food; warnings about false teachers and self-ignorance; and of course yoga instruction.

WOMEN IN THE UPANISHADS

We don't find many women in the Upanishads, but there are two named in the *Brihad Aranyaka Upanishad*. The first is Maitreyi ("Friendly"), a "scholar of ancient lore" (BU 4.5.1) and wife of the sage

Yajnavalkya (*yajna*, "sacrifice" + *valkya*, "speaker," i.e., Speaker of the Sacrifice). We meet her as her husband is readying to leave their home to become a *samnyasin*, a "renouncer." He asks her what she wants as a "settlement," presumably monetary, and she wisely asks, "If I had the whole world filled with riches, would I become immortal?" Yajnavalkya's reply is a no-brainer, the Sanskrit equivalent of, "Nope." So instead of money, Maitreyi requests her husband's spiritual knowledge, which she expects will bring her immortality. You can find this teaching beginning at *Brihad Aranyaka Upanishad* 2.4 (and repeated at *Brihad Aranyaka Upanishad* 4.5).

The second woman is Gargi Vacaknavi (from *vacaknu*, "talkative, loquacious, eloquent"), whom we find in a group of men questioning Yajnavalkya on a variety of spiritual subjects (the text doesn't explain how she ended up in this group). She asks a series of questions but is finally told she's asking too many, and warned if she continues, her "head will split open" (none of the men are similarly silenced). You can read her first exchange with Yajnavalkya beginning at *Brihad Aranyaka Upanishad* 3.6, her second at *Brihad Aranyaka Upanishad* 3.8.

» *Why don't we know the names of the men who actually wrote the Upanishads (or, for that matter, many of the old Hatha Yoga texts)?*

Nowadays it's pretty much unthinkable that an author would leave his or her name off of even the most modest literary effort (though there have been times when, reading the published version of something I'd written, I sincerely wished my name *wasn't* attached to it). I once heard or read (and now despite searching exhaustively with Google, am unable to discover its source) that even those who write books in praise of humility make sure his or her name is on the title page. For most writers, or at least the writers I know, writing is hard work, harder than anyone who isn't a writer can imagine. So it's only natural that we crave some recognition for our accomplishment, if only so the publisher knows where to mail the royalty checks.

But things were different in ancient India. The yogis who wrote the Upanishads and other sacred texts were indifferent to revealing anything about their personal lives for posterity, even to the point of evasion. Professor M. Hiriyanna ascribes this to the "humble sense which those great men had of themselves,"[19] along with their willingness to contribute to the teaching as a whole without "claiming credit for their share in developing it."[20] The result is that many of the old yoga texts reflect a group effort over many years, even generations; a foundation was laid by a single individual, and this was then added to by numerous other teachers.

» Why were the traditional teachings kept a secret?

The science of Hatha should be kept top secret (*param gopya*) by the yogi who wants success. It is powerful (*virya*) when hidden and powerless when revealed.

Hatha Yoga Pradipika 1.11

Nowadays most folks in this country, if they have a mind to, can get some yoga instruction, either in a class or from a DVD or CD, or through an online service. This ease of access is a fairly recent development, and one of the really best things about modern yoga is its inclusiveness: all can participate, regardless of gender, age, or physical condition.

This of course hasn't always been the case. Not all that long ago yoga was primarily confined to a relatively small group of mostly male initiates whose lives were completely dedicated to the practice. What's more, not only was the yoga community limited and male, but also it was highly secretive. As we read in the verse from the *Hatha Yoga Pradipika* that begins this section, the yogi is enjoined to keep what he knows close to the vest. Notice that the verse number indicates that it appears early in the text—it's number eleven out of a total of 389 verses—just after the compiler Svatmarama's brief introduction and the run-down of the masters in his lineage starting with Shiva. This surely emphasizes the importance given to secrecy by Svatmarama. In fact he enjoins his students to secrecy six more times (at 2.23, 32; 3.9, 18, 30; 4.17; and a seventh by implication at 4.2), and at least once in each of the remaining three chapters he urges discretion, not only for yoga in general but for specific practices like the ten mudras described in chapter 3 and the "Great Seal" (*maha mudra*).

Secrecy goes back to the origins of Indian yoga—in fact even beyond that, to the roots of Hindu spirituality in the *Rig Veda*. The Brahmin priests guarded the *Rig Veda*'s secrecy jealously in two rather ingenious ways: one, they restricted access to Sanskrit, refusing to teach it to anyone not in with the "in crowd" (and threatening severe punishments if outcastes even heard the language being spoken); and two, by orally passing along the mantras from one generation to the next. For a long time they did this out of necessity, since there was no writing in India. But even after writing developed, they refused at first to write down the *Rig Veda*'s mantra, rightly fearing that it was much easier for an unauthorized person to get hold of a book than the brain of a Brahmin priest.

The secret was revealed generally only to the initiated, those who had proven themselves worthy of the teaching, and perhaps the teacher's son (there's no mention of enlightening a daughter). What exactly would happen to a teacher who spilled the beans to an unqualified person? Well, the *Brahma Vidya Upanishad* (v. 47) pulls no punches: it sends the offender straight to hell.

Why were the teachings secreted from the general public? We can speculate there were at least three reasons:

1. It was believed that secrecy amplified the student's transformative energy. Like a stone rolling downhill, the student picked up momentum as his practice progressed, as long as he kept it to himself. To tell others about his secret dissipated that energy.
2. It was believed that the secret created an emotional bond among the initiates, setting them apart from those not in the know, which kept them focused on their practice.
3. The teaching was thought to invest the yogi with enormous, even superhuman, power, which in the wrong hands could be abused or misused and cause serious harm to himself and others. The best example we have of this in modern mythology is Anakin Skywalker, whose teacher ignored the warning not to train him as a Jedi (jogi?), with disastrous consequences.

Instead of heading down to the corner yoga studio for your weekly ninety-minute class, you had to *prove* your worthiness to receive the teachings. But more, you had to be ready to renounce your entire lifestyle, to chuck away your family and friends and commit yourself unreservedly to yoga. And even if you felt willing, there still weren't any guarantees that your willingness would be translated into instruction. Teachers were known to be difficult to approach and satisfy, and getting the teaching out of them was like pulling teeth—your own.

» *What is Vedanta?*

Every school of yoga has two broad elements it can't do without, a theory and a practice. The former includes a particular way of looking at the world (a "worldview"), which is usually set up in one of three ways:

1. The theory can be "one"—that is, everything in the world, from a single atom to the immense galaxies sailing majestically through space, can be traced back to a single source; this is known as *monism* (from Greek *mono*, "one, alone").
2. It can be "two"—that is, everything in the universe, from our lonely atom to our countless galaxies, has a split personality made up of two exactly opposite principles or qualities; this is *dualism* (from Latin *duo*, "two").
3. It can be both one and two at the same time—the "two" being the diverse expression of the "one," and the "one" the unifying heart and soul of the "two."

We'll meet a dualist school in Chapter 4, called Classical or Raja or Patanjali Yoga, which is based on the teaching of the *Yoga Sutra*. The focus of this chapter is on the monist school (also called nondualist), Vedanta. Vedanta is probably the most popular school of philosophy (or, if you prefer, theology) in modern India, and has been from at least the late nineteenth century. Its main source books are generally accepted to be the ten to fourteen principal Upanishads; the *Vedanta Sutra* (also known as the *Brahma Sutra*), dated sometime in the second century B.C.E.; and the venerable *Bhagavad Gita,* the date of which is up for grabs, depending on what agenda you're trying to advance (for now we'll put it sometime within 500 to 400 B.C.E., though be prepared to be contradicted by this or that scholar who wants it a hundred years earlier or one or two hundred years later).

Like most everything else about Indian philosophy, there's no simple way to describe Vedanta, especially since it's fractured over the centuries into three (that I know of) spatting sub-schools, one of which is actually dualist. So whatever I write about Vedanta will need to be taken with at least one grain of salt.

The name *vedanta* means the "end" (*anta*) of the Veda, a reference to the Upanishads. This has both a literal and a figurative interpretation based on the placement and content of the texts in question. Since they were composed after all the other texts in their line—that is, the four samhitas, the Brahmanas, and the Aranyakas—and positioned accordingly, the Upanishads are then the literal end of the Veda. But more than this, they're also credited as being the "end" or culmination of the teaching of the Veda. This conclusion isn't accepted by everyone. As we have seen, some Western scholars believe that the teaching of the Upanishads is "spiritual," while the contents of the *Rig Veda* and its offshoots are more like primitive nature poetry. Of course this incenses the Vedic traditionalists who insist there's a hidden "spiritual" message in every one of the *suktas*, and back and forth the two sides go.

So what is monism? As I suggested at the outset, monism posits a single source or Reality for the entire world. This is usually called *Brahman*, a word rooted in *brih*, "to grow" or "to expand," and which is rendered into English as "the Absolute." Technically, Brahman has two aspects, one totally passive, the other active. We might compare the latter to a painter who uses the former as its canvas. The active Brahman's power is usually called *maya* ("she who measures"), and the nature of the world she creates is a subject of some debate. Both sides in this debate acknowledge Brahman to be the only ultimate Reality. One side, let's call them the "relativists," grants the world a provisional or relatively "real" existence. The other side, however, the "illusionists," considers the world a chimera, no more than the "play" (*lilas*) of *maya*, who tricks us into thinking all the teeming diversity around us is "real," distracting us from the truth that Brahman is the one and only existent. Why *maya* wants to do this to us isn't clear to me—maybe she's just out to have a good time. But when through practice we see through this little game and reject the world entirely, poof!, it all goes up in smoke and we find ourselves absorbed back into the bosom of Brahman.

I'll let you make up your own mind about this, but personally this outlook just isn't my cup of tea. I kind of enjoy being in the play, strutting and fretting my hour upon the stage, but that just might be an indication of the depth of my attachment and ignorance. I do agree, however, with Vedanta that my consciousness and the consciousness that supports the world are birds of a feather—that is, put in Vedantic terms, *tat tvam asi*, "I am That."

4

THREADS

What Is the *Yoga Sutra*?

FOR A TIME WHEN I WAS growing up, I developed a keen interest in stargazing and wanted nothing more in life than to someday be an astronomer. That didn't quite work out as I had hoped, but somewhere along the way I learned a helpful mnemonic device, which consisted of a fractured sentence that went **M**an **V**ery **E**arly **M**ade **J**ars **S**erve **U**seful **N**eeds **P**eriod. You'll notice that I've CAPITALIZED and **bolded** the first letter of each word to give them emphasis, because they're also the first letters of the names of the planets in physical order from the Sun beginning with Mercury. Unfortunately the sentence no longer ends with a Period, since Pluto has been downsized, leaving Neptune hanging at the sentence's end.

I bring this up here because the subject of the current chapter, the *Yoga Sutra*, is a collection of similar memory aids, called *sutras*, a word that literally means "threads" (and is derived from *siv*, "to sew," from which we get the word "suture"). A collection of such threads (there are 195 in most editions of the *Yoga Sutra*, though some include 196) is often compared to a necklace on which are "threaded" the text's "pearls of wisdom."

ON THE TITLE *YOGA SUTRA*

Most translations/commentaries of the text under consideration are titled the *Yoga Sutras*, the latter word pluralized as it would be in English with an s. This seems quite natural to us, but technically it's incorrect. For one thing, Sanskrit words aren't pluralized with an s; for another, and more to the point here, a *sutra* names both the individual verse and the book that "strings" these verses together. Properly then, the basic title of the text is the *Yoga Sutra* (see, e.g., Barbara Stoler Miller's subtitle—"The *Yoga Sutra* Attributed to Patanjali"—in her translation of the work). Since this looks and sounds somewhat awkward to us, a few translators work around the situation by hyphenating the s, as in "*Yoga Sutra*-s" (see T. K. V. Desikachar's translation), which makes the title more palatable for English readers while respecting the original Sanskrit.

There are also a few translations in which the words "Yoga" and "Sutra" are hyphenated, as in *Yoga-Sutra* (see translations by Dr. Feuerstein and Chip Hartranft). This is yet another tip of the cap to proper Sanskrit. It reminds us that the two words shouldn't be separated— and that in Sanskrit the title would look like this: *Yogasutra*. Of course if we want to go completely overboard, the first letter shouldn't be capitalized, as there are no capitals in Sanskrit. This leaves us with the title *yogasutra*.

The sutra genre was popular in Indian literature from about the sixth or seventh centuries B.C.E. to about the third century C.E. A sutra has been described in many ways, for example, as a "terse aphorism" (Feuerstein), a "condensed mnemonic verse" (Hartranft), "terse and pithy philosophical statement" (Bryant), "abbreviated aphorism" (Larson), and "minimalist aphorism" (Stoler Miller). What each of these scholars is trying to convey is the extreme succinctness of each sutra, a succinctness carried oftentimes to the point of incomprehensibility.

SUTRA AS APHORISM

I certainly don't want to contradict any of the above scholars, but I would avoid comparing a sutra to an "aphorism." Although it's true that a sutra is typically a short, "pithy" phrase, nonetheless an aphorism stands on its own and clearly expresses the truth of an idea or sentiment. Most sutras simply don't; they typically need some kind of commentary to get at the implied truth. The great Indian philosopher Surendranath Dasgupta wrote that:

> The systematic treatises were written in short and pregnant half-sentences (*sutras*) which did not elaborate the subject in detail, but served only to hold before the reader the lost threads of memory of elaborate disquisitions with which he was already thoroughly acquainted. It seems, therefore, that these pithy half-sentences were like lecture hints.[1]

In other words, sutra texts aren't teaching manuals equivalent to the ones we have today, in which the teacher tries to be as detailed as possible so that the described practice stands on its own, and the student needs no further assistance or elaboration. By itself, a sutra text might be compared to the bones of a skeleton. It constitutes the framework of a system that needs "fleshing out" by either a written commentary or the oral instruction of an experienced teacher. The "viewpoint" (*darshana*, see Chapter 1) outlined in the *Yoga Sutra*, which represents the first attempt to systematize the practice of yoga, is informally called by several different names, such as Classical Yoga, Raja Yoga (see the famous translation/commentary by Swami Vivekananda), and Patanjali Yoga (after the compiler of the text).

It's curious to me that the *Yoga Sutra* has gained the kind of widespread interest it has in the American yoga community. How much interest is there? Out of curiosity, I made an informal survey of the translations/commentaries published from 1852 (the year of the publication of the first English translation) to the present. For the 118 years prior to 1970, there were twenty-five translations (that I found); in the years since 1970, I counted eighty-eight translations, more than a third of those (thirty-two) appearing in the last ten years. The appearance of all these translations suggests there's a need that exists, and scholars and teachers are more than happy to write and publish books to fill that need.

My surprise stems, I suppose, from the incongruity between the text's teaching, which describes a kind of self-absorbed, intense meditation, and the typical content of most U.S. yoga-training programs, which spend probably half of their time on detailing and refining asanas. Patanjali, in contrast, dedicates only three of 195 sutras to the subject of asanas, by which is meant nothing more than a "steady and comfortable" (*sthira sukham,* YS 2.46) "seat" (the literal meaning of *asana*) that prepares the yogi for meditation.

Still, as the first complete yoga system we have on record, there's no question in my mind that the *Yoga Sutra* is an important historical document in the development of the yoga tradition, and should have a place in any training program. Moreover, while many of its practices, if interpreted as the original teaching intended (or at least as scholars believe they were intended), may no longer appeal to modern students, the sutra genre is quite malleable, which allows innovative and enterprising teachers to interpret the text in ways that make it relevant and useful to modern students.

» *I'm reading the* Yoga Sutra *for the first time. What does it mean by* avidya? *How does that lead to suffering? Explain please.*

Recall that *avidya* is rooted in *vid,* which simply means "to know." When we put the prefix *a-* in front of it, then *vid* is turned around to mean "not-to-know" (because *a,* in one of its senses, means "not," the Sanskrit equivalent of our *un-* or *in-*).

Translators have tried out different ways to render *avidya* into English, though it's not uncommon to run across translations that simply leave it in Sanskrit. This tells us the translator believes there's no adequate way to "English-up" the word, and any attempt to do so would only muddy the waters.

But among those who do translate the term, about a third to a half of them use "ignorance." We have to be careful with this word, however, because it carries some unflattering connotations. First, when people hear or read that they're "ignorant" they tend to think that it's a comment on their level of intelligence or lack of education, whereas *avidya* has nothing whatsoever to do with either. Second, "ignorance" suggests that what's lacking is some kind of knowledge. This, again, is way off base. If we do decide to use "ignorance" then, it would be best to qualify it as ignorance of a special "spiritual" variety.

Although it's much less common, one good alternative rendering, if you have a dictionary handy, is the more academic "nescience." Etymologically speaking it's much the same as *avidya*, that is, *ne*, "not" + *scire*, "to know."

So what exactly is it that we don't know, or put another way, what is it that we think we know but couldn't be more wrong about? Patanjali's answer is in *Yoga Sutra* 2.5: *avidya* is nothing more than a case of mistaken identity or, perhaps, amnesia.

To Patanjali, our true Self has just three distinguishing characteristics. First, it's eternal (*nitya*) and so unlimited in and by time; the Self, in other words, was never born and will never die. Second, it's "pure" (*shuci*), which in this sense means it's not mixed with anything else. Just as 24-carat gold is pure gold, the Self is pure consciousness (*cit*) and nothing else. Last, because it's completely self-contained and self-sufficient without a care in the world, the Self is joyful (*sukha*). I might add here that, unlike matter, which is in continual flux, the Self is static, forever unmoving and unchanging.

Though it may seem far-fetched (and perhaps not entirely appealing), Patanjali assures us this is who we are, our true Self. Flip all this on its head and we have our mistaken self (please be aware as you read this of the difference between Self and self). The latter is, first, limited in and by time, in other words, it's ephemeral (*anitya*). I don't know about you, but the older I get the more aware I become of my own mortality, though in all honesty I can't quite wrap my brain around the inevitability of my own demise. In the end there's no denying that one day, hopefully far into the future, this self will pass away, though I can take some solace that "my" Self will not.

The self is also "impure" (*ashuci*; note how the words used to name the Self's eternality and purity are negated for the self by adding the prefix *a*- "not"). While the Self is, I guess we can say, homogenous, the self, like all material things (which includes everything there is that's not the Self), is composed of three elements, called *gunas* (known individually as *sattva*, *rajas*, and *tamas*, more on these soon). *Guna* literally means "strand" or "thread," so matter in Classical Yoga is often compared to a "rope" of the three "strands" twined about each other. What's important to remember right now is, as I mentioned just before, the *gunas* are never at rest. So while the Self is forever static and always itself and nothing else, matter is always in constant movement, constant transformation.

Finally, the self is sorrowful (*duhkha*). Understand that this sorrow isn't simply what we might experience over a broken relationship or our favorite yoga teacher moving to another city. Patanjali's sorrow is what the metaphysicians call ontological, which means that it's inherent in the nature of the world. To be alive and associated with nature (or matter) is unavoidably sorrowful, and the more sensitive we become through our yoga practice, the more intensely we experience that sorrow (I'd like to make sure it's clear that this is Patanjali's take on the world, and not mine). Though I think a lot of people will disagree with this assessment, my feeling is that, according to Classical Yoga, in order to be entirely free of sorrow, we must sever all connection to matter. Within the system, this is known as *kaivalya*, "aloneness," though we commonly know it as "death."

Avidya then is the broadly mistaken belief we all have that our self is something other than what it actually is. Why we fall into this trap isn't explained, at least to my satisfaction. Are we all simply born with the *avidya* program preinstalled in our being, just like Apple preinstalled some programs on my iPad that I don't want but can't get rid of? Apparently so, at least that's the idea I get from Patanjali.

How does *avidya* play out? Through its four accomplices, which along with *avidya* are collectively known as the "afflictions" (*klesha*). The first is "I-am-ness" (*asmita*). As I just mentioned, *avidya* is an innate tendency to misidentify who we are. *Asmita* then seals the deal by confusing the Self (*cit*) with the self (*citta*). This causes us to imagine—need I add here, mistakenly?—that each of us is an isolated individual, cut off and so alienated from all other individuals.

The next two afflictions seem to naturally pair up, one the horse, the other the carriage. The static Self needs nothing and wants nothing, it's perfectly self-contained and so quite joyous. The limited self, however, has countless needs and wants, and tries to hold on tight to what pleases it in life (*raga*, literally "to be colored," but usually rendered as "attachment") and totally avoid what doesn't (*dvesha*, "hatred, repugnance").

You may have noticed, based on your own experience over the years, that both is impossible, the good is always pulling out of the station way too soon, departing for parts unknown, however hard we try to derail the train, while the bad arrives periodically, unbidden and unwanted, at our doorstep.

I want to make sure it's clear that what I've been describing in this section is Classical Yoga's position, not mine. To my mind, a little bit of spiritual ignorance and a healthy individuality are good things if held in the right way. They can encourage and inspire us to be curious about ourselves and the world, so that we come to realize the Self not by dumping the world but by inhabiting it fully and finding the Self in the world.

» *Who was Patanjali?*

I salute Patanjali, that most excellent of sages, with folded hands. He removed the impurities of consciousness through yoga, of speech through grammar, and of the body through medicine. His upper body has a human shape, he holds a conch, a disc, and a sword, and he's crowned by a white thousand-headed serpent. I bow down to Patanjali.

KING BHOJA, from the *Commentary of the Sun King*
(*Raja Martandavritti*), ca. 1050 C.E.

He [Patanjali] is held as the author of the basic text of the School, called the *Yoga-sutra,* but is as a person perfectly legendary. Neither about his time nor about his place, anything reliable is known.

ERICH FRAUWALLNER, *History of Indian Philosophy* (1973), p. 225

As with other names associated with traditional yoga texts, like Matsyendra and the *Matsyendra Samhita* and Gheranda and the *Gheranda Samhita*, the life story of the person behind the *Yoga Sutra* is a complete blank, or at least nearly so. Since yogis and scholars disagree on the date of the *Yoga Sutra*, it's also difficult to say exactly when he might have lived, but we can "narrow" it down to the five hundred years between the yogis' preferred date for the *Yoga Sutra* of 200 B.C.E. and the scholars' estimate of 300 C.E.

DATING THE *YOGA SUTRA*

Why is there such a wide gap between these dates for the *Yoga Sutra*? One reason is that an Indian author of the time, in order to gain widespread acceptance for his work and surround it with an air of authority, would often ascribe his work to a predecessor, an expert who possessed an unassailable reputation. As we'll soon see with Vyasa, some of these "experts" acquired lifespans of hundreds, even thousands of years.

> Whatever seems good, true and right, to the Indian, that he raises to the greatest possible age; and if he wants to impart a special sanctity to any doctrine, or if he wishes that his work shall be as widespread as possible, and gain respect, then he veils his name in a modest incognito, and mentions some ancient sage as the author of the book.[2]

While nothing concrete is known about Patanjali's life, as with many of the world's heroes and holy men, a number of tall tales have attached themselves to him. One in particular concerns his miraculous birth, though it comes in at least three different versions. The most popular account involves an aged, childless yogini, Gonika, who one day wishes for a son to whom she can pass along her wisdom. As luck would have it, right at that moment the giant, thousand-headed serpent king, Remainder (*shesha*), also known as Infinite or Endless (*ananta*), was considering possible ways and means to incarnate in the human world. Taking advantage of this open door, he jumped or "fell" (*pat*) out of his heavenly realm and, in the form of a tiny serpent, landed in Gonika's joined, upturned, open palms (a reverential gesture called *anjali mudra*). The baby serpent soon assumed a human form and was named—what else?—Patanjali.

One alternative explanation for the name "Patanjali" interprets the *anjali* gesture in a much different way. Instead of Gonika's open hands being a landing zone for a sky-diving serpent, they are *patantah anjalayah yasmai*, "who the hands are folded for as a gesture of reverence."

PATANJALI AND THE SERPENT

How did Patanjali come to be associated with a giant snake? Swami Veda Bharati believes that the "greatest teacher of yoga . . . can be no other than a master of the snake called *kundalini*, which is, in fact, the snake of eternity."[3] This doesn't seem beyond the bounds of possibility, until (and here I mean no disrespect to the Swami) we bump up against two major road blocks: first, Patanjali's latest date is around 300 C.E., but according to Dr. Feuerstein, kundalini wasn't elaborated "into a full-fledged conceptual model"[4] until around two hundred years later. Second, Professor Edwin Bryant traces the earliest appearance of the Patanjali Invocation to a commentary on the *Yoga Sutra* assigned to the eleventh century C.E.,[5] at least seven hundred years after Patanjali's latest date. It doesn't seem likely then that Patanjali had any knowledge of the "serpent power" (see Chapter 5 for more on Kundalini), and that his connection with it was made long after he had left his body. Nevertheless, he's often accorded semi-divine status as an incarnation of the serpent king Shesha-Ananta and represented with a human head and torso and a lower body coiled like a snake.

» *Was Patanjali the author of two other books?*

Traditionalists assert that Patanjali was responsible for two other books, a commentary on an important Sanskrit grammar, and a treatise on India's native system of medicine, Ayurveda, literally the "knowledge or science of health." They credit him then with being an early holistic healer, providing medicine for the body, grammar (as a kind of logic) for the mind, and yoga for the self. But not everyone agrees that Patanjali had a hand in this pair of books, and that idea has given rise to good deal of heated controversy.

Based on a laundry list of evidence both pro and con, and much too arcane to go into here, we can place the participants in the debate into one of three positions that can be summarized briefly as: He Did, He Didn't, and We Can't Be Sure. Perhaps Professor Edwin Bryant has the most politic response to the question, writing that "there is not much to be gained by challenging the evidence of traditional accounts in the absence of evidence to the contrary that is uncontroversial or at least adequately compelling."[6]

It may seem strange to us Westerners that so little is known about a person of Patanjali's stature and widespread influence. If he were alive today, he might be jetting all over the world, offering weekend workshops in Raja Yoga and teacher-training intensives. But anonymity, as I mentioned above, is typical of the great sages of the East, who surely were genuinely humble people. They believed that their teaching was the "fruit" of an unselfish collective effort made over many generations, and that the individual was only a small link in this great chain.

Whoever he was, it's important to remember that Patanjali isn't the *author* of the *Yoga Sutra,* he's rather the text's *compiler.* The material he gathered together and systematized in this book, the first time that a yoga practice had been outlined in such detail, existed for a long time before him, no doubt orally, like the suktas of the *Rig Veda.*

Scholars wonder if Patanjali made any original contributions to the book, but it's nearly impossible to come to any clear-cut conclusion. Dr. Feuerstein speculates that the material for the eight-limb practice (*ashta anga yoga,* 2.28–3.35), which is by far the best known practice in the text, is a long quote from another source, and that the Kriya Yoga section (YS 2.1–27), the "yoga of [ritual] action," belongs to Patanjali. Thus, Dr. Feuerstein writes, "it is certainly one of the curious vicissitudes of history that today Patanjali's name should be so consistently associated with the 'eight-fold' path and not with the philosophically grounded Kriya-Yoga originally developed by him."[7]

» *Who was Vyasa?*

Life, as most everyone I'm sure is well aware, sometimes isn't fair. When it comes to the *Yoga Sutra,* the lion's share of attention nowadays goes to

Patanjali, the text's compiler. The *Yoga Sutra* is, as the title reveals, a sutra text. Sutra texts belong to a specific genre in Indian literature, popular from about the sixth or seventh centuries B.C.E. to about the third century C.E. But because the sutra genre is so laconic, the texts are more or less incomprehensible without an accompanying commentary by someone well versed in their teaching. Any serious study of the *Yoga Sutra* then should ideally include a close reading of the earliest commentary (*bhashya*) we have (or at least the earliest that's survived), which has exerted an enormous influence on later commentators. It was written by Vyasa, which means "arranger" or "compiler." With a moniker like that, we might reasonably expect he made his reputation pulling things together from here and there and putting them in order, which indeed is the case.

Just as with Patanjali, there's some doubt about Vyasa's identity. And no wonder. Traditionalists credit him with at least four major literary contributions, overlooking or ignoring the fact that the first and last of these efforts are at least 2,500 years apart. He started his career, the story goes, with a major undertaking, dividing the originally single text of the Veda (see Chapter 3) into four texts, for which he earned the honorific title Veda Vyasa.

As he busied himself with this chore, he labored over various accounts of the world's creation, dissolution, and subsequent re-creation, fashioning them into stories and legends of gods, kings, and warriors, and genealogies of royal dynasties—in other words, a real grab bag of tales. The contents of this bubbling stew were eventually distributed among eighteen texts collectively known as the Puranas ("ancient [tales]"), with individual names like the *Brahma Purana* or *Vishnu Purana*. Together they comprise a wildly imaginative encyclopedia, highly revered in India. Dating the *Puranas* with any degree of accuracy is nigh impossible—like many old Indian texts, they are the result of centuries of accretion—but some of the material can be traced back to at least 800 B.C.E.

Vyasa's next writing project has a backstory. While we may not know much about the historical Vyasa, his mythic biography is very detailed. He was the son of Parasara ("Destroyer"), a sage, and Satyavati ("Truthful One"), a fisher woman who was also the daughter of a nymph (he was also thought to be a partial incarnation of Vishnu). After bearing Vyasa, Satyavati regained her virginity and later married King Shantanu

("Auspicious Form"), with whom she had two sons, both of whom later married but died childless. Though Vyasa preferred an ascetic life, because of his mother's request and his social duty, he married the widows of his stepbrothers and fathered a son with each.

Apparently the women were not especially pleased with their common husband, who, according to reports, had a rather unappealing appearance. During their conjugal relations, one kept her eyes shut tight, the other turned pale with fear. As a result, one son, Dhritarastra ("Firm Empire"), was born blind, the other, Pandu ("White"), as his name suggests, was born with unusually light skin. Eventually Vyasa's two sons had a falling out, which ended, as these things often do, in an un-civil war of epic, not to mention apocalyptic, proportions.

Vyasa is credited with writing (actually dictating to his amanuensis, the elephant-headed Ganesha) the tale of this dust-up between his grandsons, titled the *Mahabharata*, usually translated as the "Great [Story of] Bharata [i.e., India]." With its one hundred thousand verses, it's reputed to be the longest poem in the world, though its greatest claim to fame comes from a seemingly minor seven-hundred-verse section known as the *Bhagavad Gita* ("Lord's Song"), which recounts an episode that takes place on the eve of an epic battle (if any battle costing the lives of thousands of men can be considered "epic").

Finally, as already noted, Vyasas produced the oldest surviving commentary on Patanjali's *Yoga Sutra*.

It seems obvious that one individual can't have been the source of all these texts, unless we accept that Vyasa lived to an extremely ripe old age. Alain Danielou suggests a possible answer to the question of Vyasa's traditionally credited literary output, though it's admittedly a bit of a stretch for even the most malleable imagination. He proposes that "Vyasa" is the name of a "cosmic entity" who's born over and over in each world cycle as an incarnation of the divine, his only job to write down the scriptures for the upcoming age. Though he may be "manifest through distinct individuals," his "character and functions" will, as the traditionalists insist, be single. Danielou concludes:

> Vyasa . . . [exists] also in ourselves as elements of the structure of our own being, and we may very well understand that this inner aspect

is the more real one and the myths of the living Vyasa and the historical avatars are only symbols.[8]

As I've said, a sutra text was never meant to be, by itself, an instructional manual; rather, it's a kind of outline or a mnemonic device, a string or "thread" (*sutra*) of terse statements that is easily memorized. This outline then helps to organize and retain large amounts of oral information. There are two schools of thought about Patanjali, the sutras, and Vyasa. One holds that Vyasa composed the commentary sometime in the fifth century C.E. The other position, which is still largely speculative, holds that Patanjali was actually Vyasa. Professor David Gordon White points out that *vyasa* also means "editor," and it "may have been a title attributed to Patanjali by none other than himself."[9] White continues that *vyasa* might have been nothing more than a pen name Patanjali assumed to write what's called a self-commentary (*svopajnabhashya*).

» Who or what are purusha and prakṛti? What is the relationship between them?

It's easy enough to describe these two principles separately, but the relationship between them is a can of worms, since supposedly each by its own nature is entirely incompatible with the other.

Literally *purusha* means "man." Dr. Feuerstein notes in his *Yoga Sutra* translation that the term's etymology is unknown, but elsewhere he suggests that it derives from *pu* ("male") and *vrisha* ("bull"), a decidedly substantial creature that doesn't exactly spring to mind when considering the immaterial purusha. Alternatively, my Sanskrit-English dictionary relates purusha to a pair of roots, *pṛṛ*, "to fill," and *puru*, "city, town," and by extension, "body." Put these two together and purusha becomes the "man who lives inside [that is, 'fills'] the city of the body."

THE "MAN" (*PURUSHA*)

The sexist undertones of the *Yoga Sutra* aren't much discussed, and really we should cut Patanjali some slack. As a product of a male-dominated culture, he was only doing what came "naturally." But *prakṛti* (or "matter," "nature"), which is a feminine noun, is in the end perfectly disposable after being used by the "man" as a springboard to his greater glory; moreover, it's purusha's entanglement with the feminine that's the source of all the misery. However, since prakṛti is insensate and purusha has nothing with which to feel, it's not exactly clear who's doing all the suffering. Despite being a masculine noun, we'll refer to *purusha* hereafter as "it."

Since it's one of those many Sanskrit words that are hard to capture adequately in English, translators approach *purusha* from various angles. I looked through about twenty translations of the *Yoga Sutra* to see which route each one followed. About a third of the translators preferred to leave *purusha* untranslated. A few went with one of the *s*-words commonly used in English to designate the spiritual principle: "soul," "spirit," or "Self" (spelled with a capital *S*, to emphasize its divine nature and distinguish it from the mundane self). Others qualified "Self" with words like "true" or "indwelling" or "spiritual." Some translators, instead of locating *purusha* as the "person inside," chose instead to emphasize its primary function, "awareness" or "consciousness," usually qualified with the word "pure" to mark its "contentless" nature (more on this soon).

Prakṛti is rooted in *kṛ*, "to make, to do," prefixed by *pra*, "before, in front of." Literally then *prakṛti* is what "makes and places before us"— that is to say, it's the stuff out of which the entire material universe, including you and me, is created. I should note here that Classical Yoga doesn't recognize a creator, so it's hard to say how the universe got started. Like every other knotty question of this kind in Classical Yoga, the response (if you want to call it one) is, "Well, that's the way it's always been."

Purusha and prakṛti are often depicted as a rather tattered pair (they remind me a little of the two lost souls in *Waiting for Godot*), one of them unable to walk, the other unable to see. Purusha, since it is immaterial, has no means of connecting with and moving through the world, but it's conscious, while material prakṛti can act, but it's completely unconscious or insensate—in other words, it lacks innate intelligence. Purusha might be said to ride on prakṛti's shoulders, providing navigational directions while purusha supplies the motive power—if, that is, the two principles had some way to interact. According to Classical Yoga's metaphysics, however, these two have been and will be forever separate. As far as how the relationship between them works, your guess is as good as mine.

Purusha is consciousness (*cit*), though a consciousness that's very different from our everyday human consciousness (*citta*). Classical Yoga's answer to one of the great philosophical questions—what is consciousness?— seems rather odd: apparently it's a little of this and a little of that. Citta is a material process, composed of the same matter as everything else, far subtler to be sure, but material nonetheless. Thus, our citta and the world around us are simpatico, "on the same wavelength" as we say today. If I look across room at my guitar, my citta registers and assumes the shape of that instrument, and says, "I love my Martin." But without the presence of purusha, the guitar's shape would be formed in total darkness with no one "there" to perceive it. Purusha, in effect, "lights up my life." Our perception then is a cooperative act—prakṛti and purusha go hand-in-hand like the old horse-and-carriage, except how they get harnessed to each other is a mystery.

According to Classical Yoga two sets of organs play a role in our ability to perceive: the *jnana indriya,* those organs that we "know" with (the eyes, ear, nose, etc.), and *the karma indriya,* those we "act" with (the hands, feet, etc.). As you can see, these two words are compounds and share a common word, *indriya,* usually rendered as "organ" but literally meaning "belonging to Indra," the name of the Vedic gods' CEO. What this tells us is that these organs, which our poor deluded ego firmly believes belongs to "I, me, mine," are in fact in the service of Classical Yoga's Indra equivalent, *purusha.* When "I" look at "my" guitar and perceive it, what's really happening is that purusha is, as in the old Beatles' song, "looking through me."

CITTA VS. CIT

Be sure not to confuse *citta* with *cit.* The former is human consciousness, which generally always has some kind of "content," whether it be a thought or memory or feeling, or, when sleeping, a dream. The only time citta is content-less, say the yogis, is in deepest dreamless sleep (in this respect, it seems all of us can partake of purusha consciousness in ordinary life, only we can never experience it for ourselves since we're fast asleep). Cit, on the other hand, is purusha consciousness, which is transcendent and content-less, always and forever.

Patanjali describes our perceptions—the shape of the guitar, for example—as disturbance on the surface of consciousness, a disturbance technically called a *vrtti*, which basically means to "revolve" or "roll." Translators have a field day with this word, trying to find just the right nuance to relay its meaning in English. I prefer Dr. Feuerstein's "fluctuation," but some other possibilities are "modifications, thought-waves, turnings, patterning, and changing states." Vrttis come at us from two directions, not only "in" from the outside world but also "up" from the depths of our unconscious as, for example, a memory. These fluctuations lead us astray, convince us we're someone we're not, and hide from us the someone that, in truth, we are. As we read in *Yoga Sutra* 1.2, Classical Yoga is defined as the restriction of these fluctuations. To borrow another metaphor, the practice of yoga, according to *Yoga Sutra*, is like slowly wiping away the dust from a mirror so that we can at last have a clear view of our true Self. (There's actually a great deal more that is involved in Classical Yoga, but I've sown enough confusion for the time being.)

ONE OR MANY?

Scholars debate whether Classical Yoga conceives of purusha as single or multiple. Those in favor of the latter position claim that there are as many purushas as there are human beings, since if purusha were single, the liberation of one would result in the liberation of all, which obviously doesn't occur. According to this perspective, purusha is as a monad or "unit," separate not only from *prakrti* but from all other purushas as well. Other scholars (including Dr. Feuerstein) argue that there is no conclusive evidence in the sutras that Patanjali saw purusha as multiple, and therefore, in its transcendent state purusha is unified, one, single.

Both purusha and prakṛti are eternal, and the world, composed of the latter, is real, not illusory as the world is viewed in some schools of Vedanta (see Chapter 3). Since it has no consciousness of its own, prakṛti is, as I described in Chapter 1, like a big wind-up toy that mindlessly keeps going and going and going; its only function, paradoxically, is to provide the means for purusha to rid itself of the world. In contrast to purusha, which is forever unchanging, "part-less" or homogenous, and blissful, prakṛti has "parts" (the three *gunas,* see below), undergoes continuous change, and, as a result, is a source, according to Patanjali, of unremitting sorrow (*duhkha,* see YS 2.15).

Here we come to a real sticking point for me in regard to Classical Yoga. Tell me, is the world to you a place of unremitting sorrow? Is all the joy and beauty you experience in life negated because you know it will inevitably end some day? Does the simple fact that life changes from day to day result in an unavoidable sense of foreboding and doom?

Certainly there are people in this world whose circumstances, through no fault of their own, create sorrow, even unbearable suffering. But for most of us, good times and bad are all mixed up, coming and going, sometimes through our own efforts (or at least we imagine so), sometimes thanks or no thanks to others. Naturally as I noted earlier in regard to attachment and aversion, we tend to cling to the good and try our best to avoid the bad, but since change is inevitable this will only intensify our sorrow. Because no matter how hard we try to do the one or the other, inevitably we're bound to fail. But what if we just accept that to be alive is to be in the midst of change, and that sometimes the change will be welcome, and sometimes it won't. I'm not suggesting this is *easy* to do—I think we can all agree on that—but neither is it *impossible.*

» What are the gunas?

The Sanskrit *tri* is etymologically related to the English word "three." Yogis are awfully fond of numbered lists, and threes play a major role in their theology, philosophy, and metaphysics. There is the *trimurti* or "three forms" of the Absolute—the deities Brahma, Vishnu, and Shiva. Then there's the *triloka* or "three worlds" of Hell, Earth, and Heaven. Finally, there's the *tri guna* or "three strands" or forces that compose the substance of the material world. Usually they're pictured as wrapped round each other like the strands of a rope.

It's thought that the whole universe is composed of differing proportions of gunas. While they're described as separate entities, it's better to think of the gunas as waves existing on a spectrum. At one end of the spectrum is the guna named "darkness" (*tamas*), which is inertia or heaviness. Its polar opposite is *sattva*, which can't be rendered exactly into English, but is defined variously as "being, existence, [spiritual] essence, purity, goodness, wisdom, consciousness." Sattva is the aspect of matter closest in nature to the immaterial Self. The motive force behind these two gunas is a third guna, "passion" (*rajas*), raw energy.

The three gunas are used to characterize and understand the make-up of natural objects or phenomena. For example, a chunk of granite is predominantly tamasic, a tornado is rajasic, and sunlight is sattvic. But what's interesting in yoga, and perhaps slightly strange to us, is that human consciousness is also considered a material process, subtle to be sure, but tangible nevertheless. This means that people's transient moods or more permanent personalities can be characterized according to the gunas. I'm sure occasionally you've felt tamasic—dark and heavy—and that you know a few intemperate human tornados, or rajasics, who never appear able to sit still and concentrate. You might even know someone who's remarkably calm and preternaturally light or insightful.

The gunas can also apply to our daily practice. Some days we're ponderous like a boulder, other days we're revved up, though maybe without much self-awareness. Then there are those rare days when we sattvically float through our practice. Traditional texts suggest that we should cultivate our sattvic nature, at the expense of tamas and rajas. This seems curious to me though. I believe it's better to cultivate a balance of the three gunas, so that, at one and the same time we're tamasically grounded to the earth, rajasically passionate about our work, and sattvically reaching for our goal, which is the realization of our authentic Self.

» What are the restraints (yama) and observances (niyama)?

Just as Jews and Christians have their behavioral do's and don'ts in the Ten Commandments and the seven heavenly virtues, so do the yogis have their behavioral admonitions in form of the "restraints" (*yama*) and "observances" (*niyama*). It's easy enough to see that these two Sanskrit words are etymologically related—both are rooted in the verb *yam*, which means "to hold or keep in, restrain, check, curb, govern, control." The restraints are generally said to regulate day-to-day relations between ourselves and others, while the observances apply to how we manage our personal lives.

The best-known examples of restraints and observances are the pentads that comprise the first two "limbs" of Patanjali's eight-limb practice (see YS 2.30–45). In popular modern commentaries they're typically presented as guidelines for our daily conduct in worldly life, and they work fairly well in that role. But I don't think that was their original purpose. The system outlined in the *Yoga Sutra* was never intended for the uplift and betterment of everyday citizens; rather, its goal was to free the solitary ascetic from what was deemed the painful trammels of worldly existence. The restraints and observances are the first baby steps in that direction, distancing the yogi from distracting entanglements with people and things, and creating a mind-set conducive to an intense regimen of meditation. Each restraint and observance, when perfected by the yogi, generates a remarkable power (described below by Vyasa). These are the five restraints:

Ahimsa (from *a*, "not," *himsa*, "hurt, mischief"). Do no harm. There are three ways to do harm: in thought, with words, and through action. Ahimsa then means to refrain from harming others not only in deed but in thought and word as well. When this restraint is perfected, you naturally disarm the minds of "living beings" around you (presumably not only humans but animals also).

Satya (literally, "real, genuine, sincere, honest, truthful, faithful, pure, virtuous, successful, effectual, valid"). Always tell the truth. When perfected, your words will be infallible or efficacious. If you say to someone, "Become virtuous," that person will immediately become so.

Asteya (from *a,* "not," *steya,* "theft"). Don't steal. When perfected, "all kind of jewels" will come to you without asking.

Brahmacharya. Literally, "moving (*car*) in Brahma" (see discussion on Chastity, below).

Aparigraha (from *a,* "not," *pari, graha,* "to seize"). Don't be greedy. When perfected, you'll be able to see into both your past and future lives.

These are the five niyamas:

Shauca. Literally, purity (see Purity, below).

Santosha (from *sam, tosha,* "contentment, joy"). Literally, contentment. When perfected, you'll acquire "unsurpassed happiness."

Tapas (literally, "heat"). Tapas is typically rendered as "austerity" or "asceticism" (see Austerity, below).

Svadhyaya (from *sva,* "self," *adhyaya,* "reading, studying"). Literally, "own reading," often rendered self-study (see Self-study, below).

Ishvara pranidhana (from *ish,* "lord," *vara,* "most excellent," and *pranidhana,* "laying on, fixing, applying; respectful conduct, attention paid to; profound religious meditation, abstract contemplation of; vehement desire; prayer"). Literally, "attention paid to the lord" (see *ishvara pranidhana*).

» *I have a friend just starting a yoga practice and so I gave her the* **Yoga Sutra** *to look at. After a week or so she came to me and asked why positive behaviors like generosity and courage aren't included among the yamas. Do you have any answer to this?*

Because the *Yoga Sutra* is one of the go-to books in teacher training programs and home-study courses, the ten behavioral guidelines that appear in the text get the lion's share of airplay. But an informal survey of a number of other books, both primary and secondary sources, turns up as many as sixty more yamas/niyamas, and it's likely that quite a few others escaped my attention and are hiding in out-of-the-way nooks and crannies. The dominant tenor of these little-known yamas and niyamas is one of balanced self-restraint, what the Buddhists call the Middle Way, wherein one walks the tightrope between the extremes of self-indulgence at one end and self-torture on the other. So we might add the following to Patanjali's list of ethical to-do's: rectitude (*arjava*), constancy (*dhriti*), resolution (*mati*), and fearlessness (*abhaya*); patience (*titiksha*), equanimity (*shama*), silence (*mauna*), and modesty (*hri*); compassion (*karuna*), sympathy (*daya*), generosity (*dana*), hospitality (*atithya*), sweetness (*madhurya*), and effort for the good of others (*para artha iha*); and finally, last but not least, bathing (*snana*). (Note that I've included in this list only those admonitions I find most pleasant, and omitted things like fasting and indifference.)

Notice we can find here the equivalents of all seven of the Catholic Church's heavenly virtues: chastity, temperance, charity, diligence, patience, kindness, and humility. We also see four of the Ten Commandments, those that forbid killing, lying, stealing, and greed or "covetousness."

But of course, if you have a list of good things to do, you probably should also have a list of not-so-good things not to do, just to make sure there are no misunderstandings. Patanjali lists nine "hindrances" (*antaraya*) (YS 1.30), which in other sources are called "obstacles" (*vigna*) and "troubles" (*upasarga*). You could probably come up with a fairly complete list simply by noting the opposites of the yamas and niyamas, so I'll just give you a few that I find especially egregious: sloth or laziness (*alasya*), boasting (*katthana*), talkativeness (*bahu alapa*), and hypocrisy (*dambha*); lust (*kama*, well, maybe a little bit is OK), pride (*mada*), arrogance (*darpa*), anger (*krodha*), greed (*lobha*), attachment (*sneha*), and jealousy (*samatsara*); doubt (*samshaya*), fear or anxiety (*bhaya*), delusion (*moha*), shame (*lajja*), dejection (*vishada*); meanness (*karpanya*) and cruelty to animals (*prani pidana*); and last but not least, that most insurmountable obstacle to any kind of spiritual progress, female companionship (*stri sanga*)—just kidding, ladies.

Not surprisingly, considering the close parallels between our yamas and niyamas and the Catholic virtues, we can find in this list all of the Church's Seven Deadly Sins: wrath, greed, sloth, pride, lust, envy, and gluttony (the yogis do indeed rail against overeating).

Now suppose you're assiduously practicing the good things and just as assiduously avoiding the not-so-good. How can you be sure you're on the right track? Just as each individual *yama* and *niyama* produces a remarkable effect, so do the practices as a group have telltale results. The inward and outward "signs" or "symptoms" that indicate success include good health and digestion; a mild manner and attractive, radiant appearance; a pleasant odor; and, best of all, a slim waist.

I have a suggestion: instead of taking on a list of pre-packaged yamas and niyamas, why not devise a list of your own, or at least supplement the traditional ten? To my list I've added generosity, hospitality, and making efforts for the good of others. How about you?

» *What is chastity* (brahmacarya)?

I think most everyone would agree that four of the five restraints seem like pretty good ideas; at least we'd be hard pressed to find anyone who is outwardly in favor of killing, lying, stealing, and greed. But the remaining restraint, *brahmacarya*—rendered variously as chastity, continence, celibacy, or abstinence—is a horse of a different color. I imagine we could find lots of people who strongly believe its flip side, sexual activity, is a terrific idea. All of the pre-twentieth-century commentators and a fair representation of modern ones don't beat about the bush when it comes to the meaning of this restraint: *brahmacarya* is *complete* abstinence from "sexual acts," no exceptions and no excuses allowed. Moreover, "acts" here isn't limited to direct physical engagement, but includes a laundry list of temptations as well; according to Rammurti Mishra, founder of the Yoga Society of New York (1958) and the Ananada Ashram (1964), it means no hearing and talking of, reading and thinking about, or watching sexual acts of any kind. He even cautions against dancing and dating if it appears likely they'll lead to any un-brahmacharya-like behavior.[10]

What's the purpose of brahmacarya in the broader yoga scheme of things? Two reasons are typically offered. Most everyone can relate to the first: sex is or can be, to a greater or lesser degree, a distraction, and the old yogis were vigilant about minimizing or eliminating anything that interfered with their practice. Second, the old yogis believed semen to be charged with an extremely potent transformative power, and went to great lengths to preserve it. They maintained that its loss sapped not only physical strength but "spiritual strength" as well. In regard to brahmacarya then, Theosophist M. N. Dvivedi (1858–1898) assures us that "No Yoga is ever reported successful without the observance of this rule as an essential preliminary."[11] How did the old yogis insulate themselves from these potential pitfalls? They went right to the source of temptation and made it their avowed policy to shun women entirely (see HYP 1.61, GS 5.26).

But times change, and some modern commentators recognize that insisting on a strict adherence to traditional brahmacarya, and the no-women interdiction, would be a tough sell to a large slice of Western students, a good three-quarters of whom are women (who, under the old system, would no doubt be warned to avoid men). So, much as was done to other practices perceived as stumbling blocks for us moderns (which we'll look at in Chapter 5), brahmacarya went under the figurative knife for a little nip and tuck. It emerged in two new and improved versions. In one, the no-way, no-how attitude toward sex becomes, instead, an honored ideal, rather than a rigid rule. If you're unable or unwilling to go the whole nine yards, then some sexual leeway is permitted, but *only* if it's responsible and appropriate. I suppose this stance is akin to what Saint Paul the Apostle proposed in his first letter to the Corinthians (7:1, 9), that it's "good for a man not to touch a woman" (and if he were living in the twenty-first century instead of the first, we can safely assume he'd add, "and vice versa"). But if you absolutely have to touch, he advised that it's "better to marry than to burn" (the King James Bible doesn't specify whether it's "with passion" or "in Hell").

The other version sidesteps the issue by steering clear of the loaded word "sex" when translating *brahmacarya* into English. Instead it relies on more neutral terms such as "moderation in all things" or "self-control." Brahmacarya, then, is presented much like meditation, as a method of focusing our usually scattered psychic energy and directing it toward the ultimate goal of Self-realization.

What happens to us when brahmacarya, at least of the traditional kind, is perfected? According to Vyasa, "strength and capacity" ensue, which "intensifies and advances unhinderable good qualities" (translation by Swami Veda Bharati), and we are then able to transfer spiritual knowledge into the minds of others.

» What is purity (shauca)?

The older forms of yoga held a decidedly negative view toward the body and the world, which is vividly, or maybe disturbingly, reflected in some of their extreme ascetic practices. Here we might recall the story of the ex-king Brhadratha and the sage Shanyana from Chapter 1. While something like the former's self-imposed ordeal doesn't seem to be part of Patanjali Yoga, the school's attitude toward the body, and indirectly the world, hasn't changed all that much since the *Maitrayaniya*. Like brahmacarya, *shauca* presents something of a public relations problem for commentators in the modern West. Patanjali instructs us to look at our body with *jugupsa*, a Sanskrit word that's impossible to paint with a happy face. "Disgust" and "aversion" are the two most common renderings; other possibilities are "dislike" and "distaste," and the off-the-charts "abhorrence." If this weren't enough, Vyasa goes a bit further. Once you lose your love for your body, he comments in *Yoga Sutra* 2.40, a "distaste develops for the company of others," and you find it impossible to come into "contact with the unclean body of another person."

Modern teachers and commentators, understandably concerned about losing their audience over this observance, try to soften the translation of *jugupsa,* with interpretations like "indifference" and "disinclination." Dr. Feuerstein counsels us to keep our "distance" from the physical, and encourages an attitude of "being on guard with respect to the body, of having a detached attitude toward our mortal frame."[12]

» What is "self-study" (svadhyaya)?

Svadhyaya is composed of four elements: *sva*, meaning "own"; *adhi*, meaning "over, from the presence of"; *ā*, "near"; and the root *ī*, "go into, contemplate." Many modern commentators, basing their interpretation on the word *sva*, take *svadhyaya* to mean "self-study," in other words, to make yourself the focus of the introspection. But this isn't exactly how this yama is traditionally construed. According to the Sanskrit dictionary, *svadhyaya* literally means to go into yourself by reciting the Veda to yourself (customarily in a low voice). I suppose this modern approach, with its emphasis on individual self-improvement, is more appealing to Western tastes than is the recitation of unfamiliar and, at times, incomprehensible ancient texts.

That said, we could conceivably adjust our practice of svadhyaya to at times include the study of ancient wisdom (and not necessarily Indian), for the truth embodied in these texts will always inspire us and bring us back to ourselves. Suggestions? Some of my favorites that aren't on most popular yoga reading lists include the *Shiva Sutra* (not to be confused with the *Shiva Samhita*), the "Heart of Recognition" (*Pratya Bhijna Hridaya*), and the "Knowledge of Bhairava" [i.e., Shiva] (*Vijnana Bhairava*).

The modern rendition of svadhyaya as self-study, however, isn't entirely inaccurate. By the study of books like the *Rig Veda*—or the Upanishads, the *Yoga Sutra*, the *Vedanta Sutra*, or the *Tao Te Ching* or Torah for that matter—the truth embodied in these texts always brings us back to ourselves. In this sense, we can say that the study of these texts then is a form of self-study.

» *What is austerity* (tapas)?

Tapas (literally "heat," from *tap*, "to give out heat, shine") is generally rendered as "austerity" or "asceticism," but we also find commentators who use terms like "self-discipline" and "mortification," which sounds rather more like medieval torture than yoga. In his study, *Tapta Marga: Asceticism and Initiation in Vedic India*, Walter Kaelber points out that, like yoga, tapas is both a "process and a product."[13] The process he calls "heated effort," and the product is "magical heat" that "saturates the practitioner, elevating him above a strictly human or profane condition."[14]

There are various ideas about what constitutes this practice. Some commentators suggest specific practices, chief among them asana and pranayama. Also mentioned are a measured diet and fasting, chastity (see Chastity, above), serving the guru (*guru seva*), seclusion and observing silence (*mauna*). Conversely Dr. Feuerstein believes that tapas "does not refer to any specific exercise but is . . . a formal category" comprised of "all those exercises which fall outside the categories of 'self-study' (*svadhyaya*) and 'devotion to the Lord' (*ishvara pranidhana*)."[15]

The *Bhagavad Gita* (17.14–16) divides tapas into three broad categories: of the body, which includes worship of the deities, the upper castes, teachers, and seers, along with the qualities of purity, honesty, continence, and nonharming; of speech, which includes self-study, and speech that is truthful, pleasant, and beneficial to others; and of the mind, which includes serenity, gentleness, silence, self-restraint, and inner purity.

» *Who or what is* Ishvara?

Ishvara is a compound of two smaller words, *ish*, "lord, master," and *vara*, "best, choicest, most excellent." Literally it means "choicest or most excellent lord or master." In most modern translations the word is either left untranslated or rendered as "God" (but we also find such sobriquets as "lord, master of life, supreme lord, ideal soul, and lord of yoga"). It's true that it can be assigned a few god-like qualities, such as omniscience and immortality; nonetheless, ishvara can't be elevated to the status of a god in the way this concept is understood in the West. Patanjali is crystal clear on this point: ishvara is a "special Self" (*purusha vishesha*) who, unlike the rest of us presumably unspecial ones, has always been and always will be in every way aloof from the world; as a consequence, it has never been troubled by the afflictions, accumulated and paid-off karmic debts, or transmigrated through multiple lives.

IT VS. HE

All of the modern commentators I researched (about twenty-five) except one refer to *ishavara* as "he." There's a real dilemma here. On the one hand, *ishvara* is a masculine noun, so technically it's proper to refer to, um, him as "he." But on the other hand, if we consider that according to all accounts, *ishvara* is attributeless, which must mean he, er, it has no gender. If this is the case, then it seems just as proper to refer to "him" as "it."

This is what's known as being on the horns of a dilemma. Should we follow the Sanskrit, or recognize the attributeless nature? I've decided, obviously, to ignore the former and honor the latter. And the one commentator who referred to ishvara as "it"? Why, one of the two women translators of the *Yoga Sutra* I have in my library, Swami Savitripriya, whose *Yoga Sutra* translation/commentary (which is quite idiosyncratic) is titled *Psychology of Mystical Awakening* (New Life Books, 1991).

» *What is* ishvara pranidhana? *(YS 2.45)*

Most commentators today render *pranidhana* as "devotion" (see, e.g., Dr. Feuerstein's *Yoga Sutra* translation, p. 42). But although the *pranidhana* entries in my two Sanskrit-English dictionaries (Monier-Williams and Arthur Macdonell's *A Practical Sanskrit Dictionary*) come close to "devotion" as a definition ("prostration, reverent salutation"), neither one spells it out directly.

If we want to think of *pranidhana* as devotion, then it's strictly a one-way street. As an unconditioned, unchanging *purusha* that has never been in contact with matter, ishvara doesn't respond to "rituals . . . or faith in his 'mercy'; but his essence instinctively 'collaborates,' as it were, with the Self that seeks emancipation through Yoga."[16] Ishvara, in other words, doesn't care a whit how much we bow and scrape at his (nonexistent) feet, and isn't concerned in the least whether our practice and its goals succeed or fail. It assists us only through its "sheer being,"[17] which provides a challenge to the yogi to emulate its nature. We might compare ishvara to a big magnet and yogis to little flecks of iron. The latter are unavoidably drawn to the former, though the former does nothing purposeful to encourage that attraction. A more accurate dictionary translation of *pranidhana* is, I believe, "abstract contemplation of."

» *Are there any asanas other than the sitting positions in the text of the* Yoga Sutra?

This is a good question and the answer is: it depends on what you consider to be "the text." In the bare bones sutra text compiled by Patanjali, asana retains its original meaning as a "seat," a simple sitting position, preferably held steady and comfortably, nothing more, nothing less. However, if you believe that Vyasa's commentary is an essential part of the teaching, then yes, there may be non-seated asanas in the text. We can't be sure of this, however, because Vyasa gives us nothing more than names, though a few are highly suggestive of modern poses.

Vyasa named eleven asanas, and we might reasonably assume that these poses were originally performed in much the same manner that they are today. They are: Lotus (*padma*), Hero (*vira*), Auspicious (*bhadra*), Mystic Cross (*svastika*), Staff (*danda*), With Support (*sopashraya*, a bound squat), Couch (*paryanka*), Heron (here called *kraunca nishadana*, the latter word means "sitting down," and is used instead of asana to denote a posture), Elephant (*hasti*), Camel (*ushtra*), and Even Standing (*sama samsthana*).

We'll look at asana in more depth in Chapter 5.

>> *The powers* (vibhuti). *I'm reading the third chapter of the* Yoga Sutra *about the yogic powers. Are they real or not? Whether they are or aren't, how do modern commentators explain them?*

Before we treat these two questions, let's take a look at the powers. Note that this section focuses only on the powers listed in the *Yoga Sutra*; additional powers are claimed for Hatha Yoga.

Of the four chapters in the *Yoga Sutra*, the third is no doubt the strangest. About three-quarters of its fifty-five sutras (which also comprise about a fifth of the total 195 sutras) are dedicated to the enumeration of the seemingly miraculous, Superman-like powers a yogi might acquire through *samyama*, the conjoint practice of concentration, meditation, and enstasy (*samadhi*). (We'll look at samyama more closely later in this chapter.) George Briggs, in his classic study, *Gorakhnath and the Kanphata Yogis*, published in 1938, writes that the "belief that such powers are attainable is very ancient, and has been held without a break down to the present day."[18]

The yogic powers are collectively known in the *Yoga Sutra* text by two names, *vibhuti* (from the verb *bhu*, "to come into being") and *siddhi* (from the verb *sidh*, "to succeed"). Each of these words has a wide variety of meanings. For example, *vibhuti*, "abundant, powerful," also refers to the ashes the yogis smear all over their bodies (see Chapter 5). It's found only once in the *Yoga Sutra*, and only in the third chapter's heading, *vibhuti pada*, usually translated as the "chapter (*pada*) on supernormal powers (*vibhuti*)." Dr. Feuerstein points out that this chapter contains material with far greater significance for yoga practice than the powers, so *vibhuti* could also be understood more broadly as *samadhi*, the state in which the powers arise.

We could go on and on with the many definitions of *siddhi*, but in regard to the powers it's usually rendered as "attainment" or "accomplishment" (and so someone who possesses such powers is a *siddha*, an "adept"). The word is found four times in the *Yoga Sutra* (2.43, 2.45, 3.37, 4.1), but only once (4.1) in reference to the powers.

Not surprisingly, the powers described in the third chapter of the *Yoga Sutra* get the lion's share of attention, yet we should remember that samyama isn't the only way to acquire them. Each of the first five limbs of the eight-limb practice (including each of the five yamas and five niyamas) have their own power-giving potential. Sutra 4.1 describes yet other means that lead to yogic powers: birth (*janman*), mantra, austerities (*tapas*), and herbs (*oshadhi*). These attract relatively little notice because they're not generally considered to be "real" yoga. Many commentators, though on the fence about mantra and austerity, are at least willing to consider these two as legitimate means, as they certainly seem to be.

But birth and herbs get raked over the coals; apparently self-realization should be slog, something earned by paying an enormous price in time and effort. So if through some karmic payoff someone is simply born to it, or finds the right concoction of, ahem, herbs to smoke, snort, or imbibe (we'll come back to this shortly), our commentators (who obviously missed the 1960s) get all huffy and dismiss any "higher" states accessed by these means as "artificial" or "inferior."

THE EIGHT "GREAT POWERS" (*MAHA-SIDDHI*)

In his commentary on *Yoga Sutra* 3.45, Vyasa lists what the yogis call the eight "great powers": (1) the power to make yourself as small as an atom (*animan*); (2) the power to make yourself light as a feather (*laghiman*); (3) the power to make yourself heavy (*mahiman*); (4) the power of reach or attainment (*prapti*), so that you can touch the moon "with a mere finger's tip"; (5) the power of irresistible will, so you can have anything you want just by wishing for it (*prakamya*); (6) the power to control all creation (*vashitva*); (7) the power to control the appearance, disappearance, and arrangement of the elements (*ishitva*); and (8) the power to manipulate the elements (*yatra kamavasayitva*).

Getting back to the samyama-related siddhis, Gerald Larson divides them into two general categories, "cognitive capacities" and "paranormal powers."[19] The former includes, among others, the intuitive understanding of the past and future (3.16), as well as our previous births (3.18) and the approach of our own death (3.22), the sounds produced by all sentient creatures (3.17), what another mind is thinking (3.19), as well as things that are subtle, hidden from view, or distant (3.25), and the composition or structure of the body (3.29).

While the cognitive capacities allow us to know things, the paranormal powers allow us to do marvelous feats or have marvelous qualities, like the ability to become invisible (21) or as strong as an elephant (24), to mindfully enter another body (38) or hear all sounds (41), to perfect our body and acquire "beauty, grace, strength, and adamantine hardness" (45–46), to master the sense organs (47), and last but not least, to fly (42).

» *I've read that the supernatural powers (siddhi) are obstacles to success in yoga. If that's true, why does the* **Yoga Sutra,** *which is supposed to value brevity of expression, devote thirty-nine verses to the subject, fully twenty percent of the total number of 195 verses?*

All authorities, including Patanjali himself, regard occult powers as the greatest stumbling blocks in the path to truth.

SWAMI PRABHAVANANDA and CHRISTOPHER ISHERWOOD,
How to Know God: The Yoga Aphorisms of Patanjali (1953), p. 181

> In India a yogin has always been considered a *mahasiddha*, a possessor of occult powers, a "magician."
>
> MIRCEA ELIADE, *Yoga: Immortality and Freedom* (1969), p. 88

Despite what they may think of them privately, in public modern-day teachers typically express a rather dim view of the supernatural powers said to develop as our yoga practice progresses. The most common objection is that they present the practitioner with mouthwatering temptations that, if bitten on, will forever poison his or her journey to the true goal of yoga, Self-realization. We might also surmise that our teachers want to distance themselves as far as possible from the powers to avoid stirring up the ire of mainstream Western religion. A good many of our priests, pastors, and rabbis are already suspicious of or downright hostile to yoga, fearing it will lure unsuspecting believers into "paganism" and so eternal damnation. There might also be a concern in the back of the teachers' minds that trumpeting yoga's bizarre powers will frighten off the more conservative members of the community and, at the same time, bring out the folks who would practice yoga not to find enlightenment or even tighter buns, but because they'd like to be invisible or read other people's minds.

It's interesting that Mr. Iyengar, though condemning the powers as a "trap," still acknowledges them as a sign that our practice is effective. "If you don't experience any of these effects," he writes, "that means your practice is imperfect."[20] His assessment seems a bit harsh. Based on it, I would venture to guess that his "imperfect" characterizes the practice of most of the estimated thirty-six million yogis in this country, including most of the Iyengar community.

A few scholars, however, point out that the powers haven't always been thought of as distractions or temptations. David Lorenzen, a scholar of religious studies, writes

> In spite of the abundant textual references to various *siddhis* in classical Yoga texts, many modern Indian scholars, and like-minded western ones as well, have seized on a single *sutra* of Patanjali (3.37) to prove that magical powers were regarded as subsidiary, even a hindrance, to final liberation and consequently not worthy of

concentrated pursuit. This attitude may have been operative in Vedantic and Buddhist circles and is now popular among practitioners imbued with the spirit of the Hindu Renaissance, but it was not the view of Patanjali and certainly not the view of mediaeval exponents of Hatha Yoga.[21]

In regard to sutra 3.37, Arthur Koestler clarifies:

> [This sutra] is the only warning in the entire text; and it only refers to certain psychic powers which are mentioned in the preceding paragraphs, whereas the powers which are listed after the warning... are held out as legitimate rewards to those who master the higher forms of contemplation. As for the later sources, the Hatha Yoga Pradipika and its companion texts, the ... siddhis are promised on practically every page. .... All disclaimers notwithstanding, the siddhis are an integral part of Yoga.[22]

» *I'm reading the* Yoga Sutra *and I'm interested in the concepts of karma and reincarnation. Could you explain something about them?*

The scene: Stan and Ollie are in Paris, where Ollie falls in love with a French beauty. But it's not to be, and Ollie, brokenhearted, decides to throw himself in the Seine and end it all. Naturally he expects Stan to jump in along with him, but Stan doesn't share Ollie's heartbreak, and doesn't want to die. There they are, standing beside the river, with big stones tied around their waists, and Stan is desperately stalling for time ...

STAN. Ollie ...

OLLIE. What?

STAN. I just thought of something. You remember once you were telling me when we passed away we'd come back on this earth in some other form, like a bird or a dog or a horse or something?

OLLIE. Oh, you mean reincarnation.

STAN. Yeah, yeah, that's it. Well, now that we're going to go, what would you like to be when you come back?

OLLIE. I don't know, I've never given it much thought. I like horses. I guess I'd like to come back as a horse. What would you like to be when you come back?

STAN. Oh, I'd rather come back as myself. I always got along swell with me.

OLLIE. You can't come back as yourself! Now come on and stop wasting my time.

From the film *The Flying Deuces* (1939) starring
Stan Laurel and Oliver Hardy

How do you view the universe? Is it, to borrow a phrase from the Roman philosopher Cicero (79–51 B.C.E.), a "fortuitous concourse of atoms," the product of pure chance? Or is it purposeful, the creation of a limitless intelligence with a master plan, however hidden from our understanding? The yogis generally fall into the latter category of believers, though the followers of Patanjali yoga hold that nature or matter (*prakṛti*) has no innate intelligence, but blindly unfolds in the "light" of the Self (*purusha*). For most yogis, the workings of the universe has an underlying purposiveness and harmony, originally called ṛta, which can be translated into something like "divine law," now known as dharma. Since we are all inhabitants of this universe, we, too, are unavoidably subject to the same rules and regulations as the planets and stars, the flora and fauna. If we can claim to have any dharma at all in these modern times, it's to play out our lives as best we can in accordance with what we can discern of the grand scheme of things.

We all have, I believe, an inborn sense of what's "right" and "proper" (two more meanings of *dharma*), what Karlfried Graf Dürckheim names (if you recall from Chapter 1) the "archetypal" or inner master, of which all the human gurus in our lives are partial embodiments. The first duty of any human guru is to help us realize our own inner guru as our constant guiding light. Be aware (and beware at the same time): any guru who encourages his or her students toward greater dependence on him or her is no guru at all.

All of our behavior, including our words and thoughts, falls under the rubric of what the yogis call *karma*. The Sanskrit word *karma* is rooted in the verb *kṛ,* which has literally dozens of meanings but can be succinctly defined for our purposes as "to do, to make." Most of us quite reasonably imagine that many of our deeds, words, and particularly our thoughts are ephemeral; once they're done, said, or thought, they have no lasting claim upon us. But no, the yogis say, everything we do, say, or think clings to us with invisible hooks, and accumulates in what's called the *karmashaya*, our own personal storehouse—or, better, bed—of *karma*. Things we do, say, or think that are more or less in accordance with dharma are feathers in our cap, are *shukla karma*, "white making or doing." Conversely, when we act in opposition to dharma—when we upset the universal applecart, so to speak—then we receive a karmic black eye, *krishna karma*, "black making or doing." Most of the time, most of us generate what we might call "grey karma," karma tinged with both white and black. So what does all of this mean?

The universe, like the human body, functions best when all of its working parts are in balance. According to the theory of karma, every one of our actions (which include words and thoughts) nudge the universe this way and that, and in order to stay on an even keel, the universe nudges us back. Our lives, in other words, are in a continual dance with karma, the white inching us along to greater and greater insight and self-knowing, the black . . . well, the black is usually accused of being the enforcer, punishing us for our misdeeds. But what purpose would that serve? I don't believe that the universe is vindictive; its goal is to always move forward toward greater and greater understanding, freedom, and fulfillment. The consequences of black karma are simply a natural result of un-dharmic behavior: If I stand and hold a twenty-five-pound weight over my foot and then let it go, the result shouldn't surprise anyone. You could say my aching foot is punishment for my foolishness, but it's also a lesson to avoid such behavior in the future.

There are two things to always remember about karma:

1. The belief is that it's good to generate good karma, and this is true *up to a point*. Good karma will influence your next birth, the quality and length of that life, so superficially your life will be relatively pleasant, though as Patanjali reminds us, whether you agree with this or not, *sarvam duhkham*, all is suffering, especially the more sensitive you become due to yoga practice. So the whole purpose of Classical Yoga is to stop generating *any* karma, and put an end to future births and suffering.

According to Patanjali, you can't do anything about what's done and past, but you can avoid repeating what's done and past by acting without attachment to thoughts and actions. This does two things: it avoids generating any new karma, and burns up the "seeds" of accumulated karma to prevent them from germinating.

In Patanjali's worldview, the ideal is to permanently detach from the "wandering through" of *samsara*, the unceasing round of birth-death-rebirth. Ultimately *any* association with matter drags on the Self and inevitably leads to some degree of suffering. The goal of Classical Yoga is, in fact, *vi-yoga*, "disunion"; what gets freed isn't the Self, which is eternally free, but a small bit of matter is returned to the cosmic matrix. In contrast, in Hatha Yoga ending our bondage to karma "Breaks the rod of Time," which means Death, and frees us to wander at will through Brahams Egg, the universe, for as long as our hearts desire (HYP 1.8–9). This is called *jivan mukti,* "embodied freedom."

2. Karma isn't fate. Our karma can be compared to a hand in a card game. We can have a pair of two's and play them well, or four aces and still play poorly. But fortunately for us, as Krishna informs Arjuna, *yogaḥ karmasu kauśalam,* "yoga is skill in performing works" (*Bhagavad Gita,* 2.50) and presumably poker.

» *I saw an ad the other day for a perfume called Samsara. Isn't that a Sanskrit word?*

It is indeed, and I wonder if the manufacturer really understands what it implies. The perfume's website says the word means "eternal rebirth" (not exactly) and is part of the "wheel of life" (and, what they don't mention, death, too). The name is supposed to evoke the "perpetual voyage from one existence to the next" (it does, sort of, but not in the way they think), which in turn is an "invitation to serenity and harmony" (it's not).

Actually, *samsara* literally means "wandering through," which already makes it seem a bit less appealing than "eternal return." In the West, I would guess the worst thing many of us can imagine happening after our demise (if we believe such a place exists) is being shipped off to the underworld. The yogis' postmortem nightmare involves a hell as well, but it's not the same as ours by any stretch of the imagination. Since the phenomenal world is, for the Classical yogi, the source of unremitting existential sorrow, the worst place he can imagine being is right here. If after passing away, he still has a karmic debt to pay, the universe will eventually kick him right back, and continue to do so until he at last can settle up and achieve Self-realization.

Gheranda compares this un-merry-go-round to a large waterwheel driven by cows, which represent our karma, and so he concludes (and we can almost hear the weariness in his voice), the embodied self (*jiva*) wanders (*bhramat*) through births (*janma*) and deaths (*mrityu*) (see GS 1.6–7). The perfume maker just might want to keep all this under his hat.

> Man in ignorance is moved like a marionette pulled by the strings of his past karmas, but a man with the help of Self-analysis takes the strings into his own hands. Man is born not only to move in the hands of karma; he is born to realize that he is the maker of karmas.
>
> R. Mishra, *Yoga Sutras*

> It [the law of karma] signifies that nothing can happen without sufficient cause in the moral as well as the physical world—that each life with all its pains and pleasures is the necessary result of the actions of past lives and becomes in its turn the cause, through its own activities, of future births. It traces all suffering eventually to ourselves and thus removes bitterness against God or our neighbor. What we have been makes us what we are.
>
> M. Hiriyanna, *Outlines of Indian Philosophy,* p. 79

I've never quite cottoned to the idea of karma. It seems to me too easy to look at people whose lives are somehow unpleasant, through no apparent fault of their own, and just shrug and say, "Well, that's their karma from a former life." I'm also unsure who, in the grand scheme of things, determines good actions from bad, and how these determinations are applied across cultures with differing values. Finally, the idea of someone claiming to be "enlightened," and so free from karma and all social strictures, seems dangerous to me, an invitation to act in any way he or she pleases and, at the same time, totally avoid any responsibility for the repercussions of those actions.

I've always valued what one my teachers once told me about karma. We're all dealt a hand of cards at birth, he said. It might be your karma or it might not, who can say? After all, your parents have their own karma, too, and so do their parents. Are we sure we're not being tainted or blessed by *their* just desserts, and not our own?

We surely have tendencies to act in certain ways, sometimes black, sometimes white, but most of us have the freedom to make a choice between the two. It may take every ounce of self-discipline you have, and you won't always be successful, but as Krishna assured Arjuna, no effort is ever wasted. But at the same time, forget all the talk of "ego-transcendence" and surrendering the "fruits" of your actions. Better to accept each one fully without any excuses. Play the hand you're dealt as best as you can. Each of us has at heart an urge to be free, and the more we give rein to that urge the easier it will be, at least in theory, to reject the black and cultivate the white for the benefit all beings, including yourself.

» *Did Patanjali advocate the use of drugs?*

The super-normal powers are the result of birth, herbs, mantra, or samadhi.

PATANJALI, *Yoga Sutra* 4.1

Yoga Sutra 4.1 doesn't get much attention in modern-day yoga. It names four alternative means by which we're able to attain the supernormal powers, listed at length in the previous chapter, that accompany the intense form of meditation known as samyama ("constraint," the conjoint practice of concentration, meditation, and samadhi, see YS 3.4). The reason for this avoidance can most likely be traced to the word *oshadhi*. More often than not it's rendered "herbs," but translators have also used words and phrases like "magical herbs," "medicinal herbs," "consecrated plants," and rarely, "drugs." Although the word "herbs" could refer to a large number of plants with a variety of uses, there's a general agreement among translators that Patanjali isn't talking about oregano for a pasta dish, but some kind of mind-altering substance, like the ancient concoction known to Vedic priests as *soma*.

This presents an interesting problem to our mostly Western translators/commentators. How will they explain what Patanjali *really* means when he *seems* to imply that we can avoid all the time-consuming, self-abnegating hassle of meditation and obtain the yogic powers simply by ingesting a fourth-century C.E. version of LSD? For many, the possibility (or should we say probability?) that Patanjali is suggesting we substitute drugs for meditation is a pretty hard pill to swallow, not least for the commentator (and his or her publisher) who would probably rather not be associated with a recommendation for drug use.

And so we're treated to some impressive interpretive spins on the word *oshadhi*. Here's how a few of our translators/commentators deal with the question:

1. Ignore it altogether, passing quickly over 4.1 to 4.2.
2. Interpret *oshadhi* as unnamed "consecrated" plants. These plants aren't in themselves hallucinogenic, so they're not really "drugs." Rather, they work because they've been ritually infused with spiritually transformative power.
3. Claim that it's the meditation practiced in previous lives that induces the extraordinary powers. (The herbs only help bring them out.)
4. Admit that, yes, drugs do have some transformative potential, but only on a much smaller scale than meditation. Drugs merely create a temporary, uncontrollable transformation; the "real" lasting transformation comes only through dedicated meditation practice. This particular response is quite old. The *Yoga Shikha Upanishad* (1.152–54) cautions that

    > Psychic powers are of two kinds in this world; artificial and unartificial. Those psychic powers that prevail by having recourse to means, such as the various ways of employing mercury and medicinal herbs, the practice of mystic spells and the like, they are known as artificial. Such powers, as arise out of the employment of the (above) means, are transient and endowed with little efficacy.

5. Attack. One translator/commentator who took this approach was Charles Johnston, a Sanskrit "prizeman" for both the Indian Civil

Service and Dublin University. In his 1912 "Introduction to Book One" of the *Yoga Sutra*, Johnston asserts that the *Yoga Sutra* "contain the essence of practical wisdom,"[23] and that the sutras are "closely knit together" and can't be "taken out of their proper setting."[24] But when he comes to 4.1 and the *oshadhi*, "practical wisdom" takes a back seat to his Christian outrage:

> Psychical powers may be gained by drugs, as poverty, shame, debasement may be gained by the self-same drugs. In their action they are baneful, cutting the man off from consciousness of the restraining power of his divine nature. . . .[25]

This is, of course, another prime example of how we Westerners interpret Indian texts and their teaching based on own biases and prejudices.

The most honest approach would be to acknowledge straight out that Indian yogis and priests have been using hallucinogens for a very long time as part of their practice and sacrificial rites. In the *Rig Veda*, for example, we can find numerous mantras extolling the use of *soma*, "nectar." Known as the "elixir of immortality," *soma* apparently was a powerful hallucinogenic concoction made from the juice pressed from a now forgotten plant, and played an essential role in the priestly ritual.

Where there are joys and pleasures,
gladness and delight,
where the desires of desire are fulfilled,
there make me immortal.
O drop of Soma, flow for Indra.

Rig Veda 9.113.11 (translation by Wendy Doniger)

In the Hatha Yoga tradition, Shiva is the "lord of hashish" (*carasa*), and many of his devotees up to the present day avidly follow his puffing lead.

What does our friend Vyasa have to say about *oshadhi*? Interestingly, he asserts that it can have a significant and positive impact on our lives. There's one catch, however. The elixir, whatever it is, can only be obtained at the "mansions of the demons" (*asura*), though no one is sure exactly where these mansions are or how to get there. But if we do happen to stumble upon them, Vyasa assures us that lovely demon damsels (which seems like a contradiction) will serve us the elixir, drinking which we attain "agelessness" and "deathlessness." This certainly seems pleasant enough to me, at least for a few centuries.

» What is samadhi *("put together")?*

The word *samadhi* is rooted in *dha*, literally "to put." When we add on the two particles, *sam* and *a,* this imposing, mystical-sounding word simply means "to put together." I was interested to see how translators and yoga commentators have interpreted this important word. In about a third of the works I consulted, they decided not to venture into deep water and left the word alone. In the remaining works, the translations were all over the map, and no two translators used the same word. Among the words that most approximate "to put together" are "absorption" (from Latin *absorbere*, "to swallow up"), concentration (from Latin *com-*, "together" + *centrum*, "center," i.e., "to center together with"), and enstasy (*en-*, "to go into" + Greek *stasis*, "standing still"). It's difficult to describe samadhi in twenty-five words or less, not only because it's a complex subject, but also because the commentarial literature on the subject is far from clear. Let me try to "put it all together" as simply as possible.

According to Classical Yoga, we're stuck in an existentially painful situation, caused by a grievous misapprehension of our true identity. We think we're a material being, limited in space, in time, and in knowledge, assaulted by, as Hamlet (3.1) says, the "heartache and the thousand natural shocks that flesh is heir to," but in fact we're not any of that at all, at least not in an ultimate sense; instead, we're an immaterial, eternal, blissed-out, um, *principle* (for lack of a better word), also known as the Self. Why this Self agreed to this most unpleasant connection with matter is anybody's guess, and why this Self finds it so difficult to extract itself from what is obviously a losing proposition is, again, a question no one seems able to answer.

Be that as it may, how does this Self free itself from such an untenable situation? The answer given by Classical Yoga is that it should undertake a program of intense meditation, in and through which it discriminates (*viveka*) between its immaterial self and this material not-self. This discrimination, in turn, leads to *vairagya,* which translators typically render as "dispassion" or "detachment." It is by this vairagya that the Self drops its material trappings and gains freedom. While the word "dispassion" may adequately relay the intent of *vairagya,* it misses the impact of the term's literal meaning, which is "growing pale." What this tells us is that we're "colored" by our materiality, and as we slough it off we grow increasingly "color-less" or translucent, until, when at last we have shed all identification with matter, including with the material body (an event otherwise known to our limited minds as "death"), the light shines through us without any hindrance.

Vairagya has a close companion, *abhyasa* (see YS 1.12). While many Sanskrit words are rendered variously into English, this is not so with *abhyasa.* Almost unanimously, the word is translated as "practice." Now "practice" is OK, it gets the basic idea across, but it's really not forceful enough. I "practice" my guitar for thirty minutes to an hour most days (not that it's doing me much good), but this level of practice won't get any significant results when it comes to Classical Yoga. In order to relay the full meaning of "practice" in the context of Classical Yoga, we need a qualifier or two, which is exactly what Patanjali gives us in *Yoga Sutra* 1.14: we must practice "assiduously" (*asevita*) and for a very long time "uninterruptedly" (*nairantarya*), in other words *all the time.*

And what is it that we're practicing so assiduously for such a very long time? Practice, says Patanjali, is the exertion or zealous effort (*yatna*) we must make to stabilize the otherwise chattering consciousness and create a state of stillness (see YS 1.13).

If matter were nothing more than what we experience with our senses, this silencing of the mind might not be such a chore. Unfortunately, there's more to matter than meets the eye. Our familiar sensory world is just the tip of the matter "iceberg." Below the "water line" is a hidden world of subtle matter that, as we penetrate into it more and more deeply, becomes more and more subtle, and so harder and harder to distinguish as "not-Self."

We obviously can't use our physical senses to enter and explore this subtle realm, especially as the difference between Self and not-Self becomes almost indistinguishable. Another strategy is needed. Since the yogi's physical senses aren't of any use, she shuts them down and internalizes the object of meditation in her consciousness. The two—that is, the object of meditation and the yogi's consciousness—are then "put together" (*samadhi*) so the yogi experiences the object directly, or we might say, in its essential nature. At this advanced stage in the meditation practice, I haven't a clue what this object may be, but it hardly matters in the end. Because regardless of what it is, even the subtlest of thoughts, it's still matter (*prakṛti*) that the yogi, with her exquisitely refined sense of discrimination (*viveka*), realizes is "not-me." With this final insight, she severs the last tenuous connection with her mistaken identity and steps into the light of her true Self (*purusha*).

This, friends, is a greatly oversimplified account of samadhi, the eighth "limb" (*anga*) of Patanjali's eight-limb practice and the penultimate state of Classical Yoga, the ultimate being what is appropriately but rather chillingly named *kaivalya*, "aloneness."

» *Since there are so many translations of the* Yoga Sutra *available, how do I know which one is best for me?*

This is a difficult question to answer. I have my favorite translations, but certainly they wouldn't all appeal to everyone. Then there are those I don't refer to much that would no doubt appeal to lots of students. In the Notes section at the end of this book, I've listed twelve volumes for your consideration. You'll find them grouped under three headings: Old Standbys, Indian scholars/teachers, and Western scholars/teachers.

5

FORCE
What Is Hatha Yoga?

>> *You've been doing yoga now for longer than I've been alive.*
What was it like to practice yoga back in the 1980s?

I have trouble remembering what I did yesterday, and you want me to re-member what it was like in 1980? Well, it was a much different yoga world back then. For one thing there were hardly any yoga schools around, un-like today when there seems to be one on every street corner, like gas sta-tions, with new ones popping up every day. The reason for this is simple supply-and-demand. Thirty-five years ago yoga wasn't the big business that it is today. A recent survey by a popular yoga magazine somehow came up with a tally of more than thirty-six million yoga practitioners in the U.S., who collectively spent an estimated twelve billion dollars—yes, that's billion with a *b*—on yoga in 2015, for everything from classes and workshops, to books, CDs and DVDs, props, vacations masquerading as "retreats," and, last but not least, yoga "togs."

Back then, class fees were under ten dollars, there were few books avail-able and no CDs or DVDs (the earliest yoga tapes were VHS cassettes), mats could be had for a few bucks (though depending on the intensity of your practice, they'd only last a couple of months at most), retreats were rare and usually hosted at rustic centers in northern California (and not in India or South America or Hawaii), and everybody, women included, wore their old baggy clothes to yoga class (not today's two-hundred-dollar "yoga uniforms"). Oh, and nobody carried water bottles into class or kept their cell phones next to their mats, just in case the President should call for advice on the crisis in the Middle East (admittedly, neither plastic water bottles nor cell phones existed back then).

In 1980 I was living in Oakland, just across the border from Berkeley, and all I knew about yoga I had learned from a brief conversation ten years earlier, on a trip two friends and I made across Canada. In Vancouver, I had struck up a conversation with a young woman on a beach, and at some point, no doubt out of boredom, she drew her feet together and sat in what I now know is Bound Angle (*baddha kona*). Then she began bobbing her knees up and down; she told me the exercise was named Butterfly. Had I known then what I know now, I might have told her that by the way she was doing the pose it should have been called the "groin tightener." Somehow I don't think that would have impressed her.

I won't go into the details of quite how it happened, but in 1980, long after this conversation, I discovered "spiritual" books: Jiddu Krishnamurti first, then Peter Ouspensky, who in turn lead me to one of his students, Robert de Ropp. I read in one of de Ropp's books that the best exercise ever invented was yoga. Then just a day or two after this "seed" was planted I saw an advertisement in a local paper for some place called the Yoga Room, which was an easy walk from my apartment. In those days, I didn't believe in messages from the universe (and I'm not sure I do now), but the coincidence seemed especially meaningful. So it was that in May of 1980 I took my first yoga class.

I had no idea what to expect, other than the bouncy-knees Butterfly. The teacher was a stocky, bearded, good-natured fellow who regaled us with stories of his trips to India and his training with an Indian teacher by the name of Iyengar. It took me awhile to figure it out—and I can't say that it was the universe at work again, since to my memory this was the *only* yoga school in the East Bay at the time—but I had unknowingly, and quite fortunately, stumbled upon an Iyengar-influenced yoga school. (You could call your yoga studio "Iyengar-influenced" back then; there was not yet an official Iyengar certification.)

The class was way, way harder than Butterfly had led me to believe. Though I wasn't in tip-top shape, I wasn't in bad shape either. Still, by the end of class I was drenched in sweat, and my limbs were heavy with fatigue. I kind of enjoyed it but kind of didn't, too. Eventually, the part of me that liked it won out and I became a regular at the Yoga Room.

After about two years, for reasons that are now long forgotten, I decided to enroll in the teacher training program at the Iyengar Yoga Institute in San Francisco. Did I have plans to become a teacher? Maybe, although thinking back to who I was then, becoming a teacher was only a shade more likely than becoming an F-16 pilot or a brain surgeon. Nowadays all of the larger yoga schools have training programs, but in 1982 the IYI program was the only game in town (in fact, in pretty much all of the West Coast; the school even attracted students from Japan and Europe).

Most programs nowadays are over and done in two hundred hours, and as a result yoga teachers are multiplying faster than Tribbles. The IYI training, however, lasted two years, and the "hard" courses—anatomy, physiology, kinesiology, and so on—required a substantial amount of study. There were no free passes: you either did the work satisfactorily or you didn't graduate. I made it through the program in about three years (and this future author of two books on pranayama earned an unremarkable B+ in one of his pranayama courses). Not long after this, the goofy guy I'd become friends with in the program came to me and said, "Hey, let's open a yoga school." I thought he was nuts, and I replied, "Rodney, you've got to be kidding." But he wasn't, and we did, but that's a story for another time.

YOGA STORY

The origin of Hatha Yoga (Version 1)

According to the earliest version of Hatha Yoga's origin (from the KJN 16.27–46), once upon a time Shiva and his beloved spouse, Shakti, traveled to Moon Island. There Shiva wrote down the sacred teaching (*agama*) of the "family" or "flock" (*kula*), called so for two reasons:

1. because in order to receive the teaching you must belong to the lineage or "flock" of initiates, and

2. the teaching's practice culminates in the union of the knower (the subject or practitioner), the known (the object of meditation), and the knowing itself, which are then related to each other like the members of a close "family."

Soon they were joined by Shiva's young son Karttikeya, whose name derives from that of his six foster mothers, the Krittikas (who form the star cluster we know as the Pleiades). Karttikeya wasn't really spiritually qualified to receive the "family" teaching—he was *ajnana,* "unknowing"—but his father transmitted it to him anyway, and the result was predictable. In a fit of pique, Karttikeya stole Shiva's sacred text (*jnana patta,* literally "tablet of knowledge") and threw it into the sea, where it was swallowed whole by a fish. Angry, Shiva went to the sea and hooked the fish, cut open its belly, and recovered the book.

Taking no chances Shiva hid the book where he believed Karttikeya couldn't find it. But his son was determined. Transforming himself into a mouse, Karttikeya (in the story here called Kruddha, "irritated, provoked") dug into the hiding place, found the book, and again threw it into the sea, where it was eaten this time by a "great fish" (*maha matsya*). Now Shiva was furious. He caught the fish in his "Shakti net," but the fish was so big and powerful that even Shiva didn't have the strength to drag him to shore. He enlisted the help of the thirty-three gods—the Rudras, the Ashvins, even Indra and Prajapati—but the fish still couldn't be conquered. Shiva decided that as a Brahmin he didn't have the necessary skills to land the fish, so he renounced his caste and assumed the persona of a fisherman. Only then was he able to capture the fish and again recover the sacred teaching. This story explains why Shiva is sometimes called the Fish Killer (*matsya ghna*).

Ultimately this secret knowledge lives in the "middle" (*madhya*) of the embodied self (*jiva atman*), and is as essential to our being as the flower (*pushpa*), root (*mula*), and fruit (*phala*) are to a plant.

» I've heard that the definition of hatha is something like "Sun-Moon." What exactly does that mean?

Ha signifies the sun and *tha* signifies the moon. The union of Sun and Moon itself is called Hathayoga.

BRAHMANANDA in his commentary (*jyotsna*)
on the *Hatha Yoga Pradipika* 1.1

It's not uncommon for a word in the yoga lexicon to have two levels of meaning, one esoteric (inner) or figurative, the other exoteric (outer) or literal. The exoteric meaning of hatha is quickly found in a Sanskrit-English dictionary. Much to the surprise of many students, hatha means "violence," "force," and "obstinacy." Literally then, Hatha Yoga is the "forceful union-method" (for the definition of yoga, see Chapter 1), with perhaps the implication that, if we expect a successful outcome to our practice (however we define "practice" and "outcome"), along with being forceful we also must be obstinate, and downward-doggedly stay on course no matter how many obstacles we encounter in our work.

Now what exactly does "force" mean in the context of traditional Hatha Yoga? I imagine that what probably comes to mind right away for us moderns when we hear that word is the teeth-gritting, eye-popping, sweat-drenched, do-or-die effort we often see in some classes, mostly among Type A yogaholics of the male persuasion.

Certainly there are times in the old books when such an extreme application of force seems to be encouraged, though other times the reverse seems to be favored. We have a good example of the former in the *Hatha Yoga Pradipika*'s (2.7–13) instructions for a preliminary breathing practice (though it's not named in the text, the practice is called "purification of the channels," *nadi shodhana*). In the first half of verse 2.9, Svatmarama instructs us to hold the inhaled breath to the limit of our capacity, which would seem to require some serious forcefulness; indeed, because of this he cautions us that at first the effort will make us sweat, probably profusely, and then tremble (2.12). But right on the heels of this, in the second half of the verse, he exhorts us to exhale the breath gradually or gently (*shanais*), never fast (*na vegata*), which seems to suggest that we shouldn't, at this time, apply excessive force. Svatmarama eventually comes down on the side of the slow-and-steady tortoise approach to practice, and he has some dire warnings for all the hares, who, speeding too rapidly to their goal, risk respiratory problems, various unspecified aches, pains, and diseases, and in the worst case scenario, death (*hanti*, "killed")—which seems a bit of an exaggeration for the purpose of getting his point across.

We find a similar volte-face in the *Gheranda Samhita* some two hundreds years or so later. In one verse (5.59), Gheranda directs his skull-bearing student Canda to retain his breath with "great effort" (*bahu yatna*), until his nails and hair start sweating. In all my years as a student even with all the superhuman efforts I've made to stay in a posture beyond the time I could reasonably be expected to survive—an experience otherwise known as Iyengar training—I don't think I ever felt my fingernails sweat. I'm not even convinced fingernails *can* sweat, but if they can and do, this to me screams "force." But twenty verses later (5.78), in describing the now forgotten pranayama called Fainting (*murccha*), Gheranda tells Canda to practice retention with "comfort" or "ease" (*sukha*).

In this first sense then, the word "force" (*hatha*) characterizes the overall practical approach of the school as "Forceful Yoga." We should keep in mind, though, that "force" is always applied as appropriate to the situation, that in some practices the application of a vigorous force is needed, while in others it should be dialed back to a minimum. Notwithstanding some of the sensationalist reports we sometimes hear of yogis performing extreme austerities, like holding one arm upraised for years at a time, or sitting in the open amid five fires in the heat of an Indian summer afternoon, when it comes to the application of force Hatha Yoga generally walks down the middle of the road.

But there's a second way that "force" has been interpreted when paired with "yoga," and this is as the mysterious force known as *kundalini*. In this sense the word, rather than characterizing the nature of the practice, tells us about its focus, that is, Yoga of the Force. We'll come back to this fascinating subject a little further along in this chapter.

So much for the exoteric definition of hatha. Now what about the esoteric? Well, it isn't found in any dictionary. It's been arrived at by taking the word *hatha* and dividing it into its constituent syllables, then assigning to each of them an arbitrary meaning that will, when combined, tell a story that supplements or amplifies the literal meaning. In the case of hatha, the first syllable, *ha,* is designated as "Sun," the second syllable, *tha,* as "Moon." These are undoubtedly very old equivalences, though just how old is difficult to estimate, given the vagaries of dating the texts. Let's leave it at several hundred years. One of the earliest (if not the earliest) instances of hatha interpreted as "Sun-Moon" is found in the *Seed of Yoga* (*Yoga Bija,* 158):

> The meaning of the term Hathayoga is pranayama sadhana. The letter *ha* in hatha signifies the flow of prana breaths in the solar [Sun or *pingala*] nadi, and the letter *tha* signifies the flow of the prana breaths in the lunar [Moon or *ida*] nadi. When the Sun and the Moon become one during the process of pranayama . . . the ignorance created due to all sorts of imperfection is removed.

Traditional Hatha Yoga is most closely identified with pranayama, not asana as it is today in Hatha Yoga's modern offshoots. This is the hidden message in "Sun-Moon." It tells us first about the two opposing (or if you prefer, complementary) subtle psychoenergetic currents (ida and pingala, Sun and Moon), signified by *ha* and *tha,* that govern our lives, and which are the focus of pranayama practice; then it hints at the goal of pranayama, which is the joining (*yoga*) of these currents in the third main energy current, the "most gracious channel" (*sushumna nadi*), also known as the "middle path" (*madhya marga*). As Svatmarama writes: "When the breath goes into the middle, a steady mind is born" (2.42), which he characterizes as *manonmani,* "mind-no mind" (4.2), a synonym for *samadhi.*

>> *I've read in several old books that Hatha Yoga is a preparation for Raja Yoga. This doesn't seem to be the case nowadays at all. Was this ever true?*

> Raja-Yoga and Hatha-Yoga are necessary counter-parts of each other . . . Hatha-Yoga deals entirely with the physical body.
>
> ALAIN, Yoga for Perfect Health (1966), p. 19

All this practice [of Hatha Yoga] is pronounced as distinctly useless . . . unless it leads to *Raja-yoga*. . . . It will thus be seen, that all kinds of *Yoga* are useful in leading to the end, *Raja-yoga*. Unless they lead to this end they are of no use whatever.

M. N. DVIVEDI, *The Yoga-Sutras of Patanjali*
(1890), pp. 129–31

Hatha yoga was designed to prepare the aspirant for spiritual experience by perfecting his body; but it has been condemned by spiritual teachers because it tends . . . to concentrate the mind upon the body itself. In the West, it is to be found in a completely degenerated form, as a cult of physical beauty.

SWAMI PRABHAVANANDA and CHRISTOPHER
ISHERWOOD, trans., *How to Know God: The Yoga Aphorisms of Patanjali* (1953), p. 69

Hatha Yoga is only the beginning of Yoga. The Yoga of the body is but a paving of the way for the Yoga of the mind.

WILLIAM ZORN, *Yoga for the Mind* (1968), p. 2

Raja Yoga includes Hatha Yoga within its system.

JAMES HEWITT, *The Complete Yoga Book* (1978), p. 9

It's not surprising to me, given the sentiment expressed in these quotes (and many others not gathered here), that so many present-day students still buy into the idea that Hatha Yoga is predominantly a physical practice and the first step in and preparation for the Raja Yoga. As B. K. S. Iyengar writes, "Those who approach yoga intellectually say that raja-yoga is spiritual and hatha-yoga merely physical. This is a tremendous misconception."[1] There are, I believe, at least two sources for this misconception.

One is the public teaching of the self-proclaimed Swami Vivekananda. His speaking tour of the U.S. in the mid-1890s, which followed his attention-grabbing presence at the World's Parliament of Religions in Chicago, gave average Americans their first taste of "yoga philosophy," at least his version of it. By the late 1800s in India, Hatha Yoga had fallen on hard times and was reviled by both respectable orthodox Hindus and their British colonizers. The British-educated Vivekananda had originally come to the U.S. to raise money for his social reform projects back home. Nowadays we're used to exotic-looking people lecturing on exotic-seeming subjects, but in the 1890s Vivekananda, with his robe and turban, must have seemed like a visitor from another planet. It was in his interest then to make the subject of his talks as non-threatening and familiar as possible, and to distance himself as far as he could from anything that would antagonize his audience. That included Hatha Yoga.

In his interpretation of and commentary on Patanjali's *Yoga Sutra*, published in 1896 and significantly titled *Raja Yoga* (*raja* means "king, best of its kind," and is cognate with our "royal"), he wrote that Hatha Yoga "deals entirely with the physical body" and doesn't "lead to much spiritual growth."[2] Since Vivekananda was one of the first individuals to talk publicly to large audiences and write books on the subject of yoga, a fair number of Americans uncritically accepted his low opinion of Hatha Yoga. This criticism persisted in some quarters, as we can see in the quotes above, all the way up to the last quarter of the twentieth century.

The other source of the misconception that Hatha Yoga is merely a stepping stone to the "higher" practices of Raja Yoga, is to be found, ironically, in one of the foundational texts of the Hatha Yoga tradition, the fifteenth-century *Hatha Yoga Pradipika*. Or to be more precise, it is the misreading or misinterpreting of this text's opening verses that has caused such a misconception to be propagated. In 1.1, Svatmarama proclaims that Hatha Yoga is a figurative "staircase" (*adhirohana*) we can climb to the penthouse of Raja Yoga. Customarily, "Raja Yoga" refers, as we see with Vivekananda's title, to Patanjali Yoga, *but not here*. If we turn to 4.3–4, we come upon a long list of sixteen terms that mean the same or nearly the same thing—in other words, they are synonyms (*eka vacaka*). And the first two entries on this list? "Raja Yoga" and "*samadhi*." Samadhi is then defined in more detail in the next three verses (4.5–7): it occurs when prana "wanes as the moon" (*kshi*), the mind dissolves (*prali*), and the embodied self is absorbed in the great Self. Clearly then, Svatmarama's staircase leads not to the "higher" practices of Patanjali but to the ultimate *spiritual* goal of Hatha Yoga and Raja Yoga both, that is, *samadhi*. Yogi Hari, who teaches something called Sampurna Yoga, the yoga of "fullness" or "completeness," sums it up: "The term *Raja Yoga* is not used here to describe a system but rather a state of consciousness. It is simply astonishing how there can be any confusion about this when the Shlokas [verses] are clear."[3]

» *I've heard that some practices of Hatha Yoga can be dangerous, especially Head Stand (shirshasana) and Shoulder Stand (sarvangasana). Is there any truth to this?*

One does not wish to put any of these hatha-yoga practices into print, to be read by various kinds of people, without sounding a warning. Many people have brought upon themselves incurable illness and even madness by practicing them without the proper conditions of body and mind.

ERNEST WOOD, *Great Systems of Yoga* (1988), pp. 90–91

There are lots of yoga teachers and physical therapists who would answer this question with an emphatic, "Yes, it's true!" The seven relatively delicate vertebrae of the cervical spine, they insist quite reasonably, are designed to bear the weight of the head, estimated to be between ten to fifteen pounds, not the weight of the body, which can be more than ten times heavier (that's the job of the cervical's five massive compatriots lower down in the lumbar spine). This anti-inversion crowd warns that repeated stress on those neck bones while holding inversions can lead to all sorts of unhappy consequences, many of them too gruesome to mention. And don't try to tell the most militant of these folks that there are ways to perform these poses that greatly diminish, if not eradicate entirely, the threat of injury. To them, standing on your head is a bad idea, period, and the poses should be summarily tossed on the Hatha Yoga trash heap, along with, say, the cutting of the frenum for *khecari mudra* (a practice that belongs firmly on the esoteric side of things).

On the other hand, there are lots of yoga teachers who reply, to the contrary, that inversions, particularly head stands and shoulder stands, can be done safely and sanely. The difference is while the anti-camp ends its argument with an uncompromising period, the pro-camp must qualify its position. The pros have to side with the antis to a certain extent, because there's no denying there are a substantial number of students who should completely avoid one or the other or both of these poses in their full-fledged, weight-bearing-on-the-neck versions (though there are ways to approximate the poses that don't put any weight on the neck, by using chairs, specially-built contraptions, or pelvic slings as supports). Raw beginners and weekend Warriors, for example, usually haven't the strength, flexibility, and sensitivity to do a full head stand, and they should be banned from its performance until they cultivate these qualities (since this isn't an instructional manual, I won't go into the nuts and bolts of teaching inversions properly).

Students aren't the only ones, by the way, who should be warned away from inversions. The countless two-hundred-hour teacher training programs around the country, many of them of questionable value, are yearly cranking out heaven knows how many brand-new teachers, all rarin' to go. Enthusiasm is a highly desirable trait in a teacher, but these novices have no business teaching inversions. They generally need additional training and more experience with a toes'-eye view of the world, before leading others into these poses.

>> *The other day I read something in one of the old Upanishads that disturbed me deeply. It was a description of the human body as "evil-smelling... afflicted with desire, anger, greed, delusion, fear, despondency, envy... old age, death, disease, grief and so on." Is this what yoga really thinks about the human body?*

The body is my temple, and asanas are my prayers.

B. K. S. IYENGAR, *Iyengar: His Life and Work* (1987), p. 495

The book you were reading is the third-century B.C.E. *Maitri Upanishad* (1.10–12), and yes, it's true that some of the teachings associated with traditional yoga have what we might characterize as a negative or pessimistic attitude toward the body (and for that matter, the world in general). (Ironically the Sanskrit *maitri* means "friendliness.") Some of the best examples of this attitude (or worst, depending on how you look at it) are found in the anthology of texts collectively called the Samnyasa Upanishads (*samnyasa*, "renunciation"). "If a man finds joy in the body," one of them says, "a heap of flesh, blood, pus . . . tendons, marrow, and bones—that fool will find joy even in hell" (*narada parivrajaka upanishad* 145). Nice, huh?

But this view of the body, and the world, is countered by later yoga texts assembled under the powerful influence of the Tantric revolution. Emerging around 800 C.E., but with roots reaching back a few centuries earlier, this movement, writes Dr. Feuerstein, viewed the world not as a "mere illusion but a manifestation of the supreme Reality." He continues that if the "world is in essence divine, so must be the body. If we must honor the world as a creation . . . of the divine Power (*shakti*), we must likewise honor the body."[4]

From the perspective of Hatha Yoga, if you're inhabiting a human body, you're necessarily the beneficiary of past good karma. However outwardly miserable your current life may be, the yogis still insist that a human body is the universe's greatest gift. So let's put the *Maitri Upanishad* back on the shelf for a moment and take down the tenth-century C.E. *Flood of Kula Tantra* (*Kularnava Tantra* 1.15, 18).

> Of the 8.4 million bodily forms, the human body is the most important, for it is this form in which one gets knowledge of the essence. . . . No creature in any other form of body than human can pursue higher aims of life. Therefore, endowed with the precious wealth of a human body one should indulge in virtuous deeds.

Feel better?

>> *In my teacher training program, we spent one of the classes talking about yoga's subtle anatomy. Could you give us your perspective on this subject?*

When a yogi looks at the world, he sees things that are completely beyond the ken of our everyday senses. We might scoff at such a claim, but at the same time we readily accept a modern astronomer's assertion that only about twenty-five percent of the stuff that makes up our universe is actually visible. The rest, what is called dark energy and dark matter, is beyond the range of even our most powerful instruments.

At this very moment, say the yogis, we're living in a world made out of both gross and subtle matter, the former of course what we see and taste and touch everyday, the latter hidden away from those senses and accessible only in states of intense meditation. We might think, moreover, that our gross universe is more "real" than the subtle, but no, say the yogis, it's just the other way around. The gross is an outpouring of the subtle, which in turn stands in the same relationship to the ultimate creative force, call it Brahma or Shakti or whatever (I don't imagine it much cares one way or the other what name we give it).

I'm not sure I understand much of this—in fact, to tell the truth, I don't understand it at all—but according to modern astronomy, at least three-quarters of the stuff that makes up the universe can't be directly seen. It's out there somewhere, it can sort of be measured, but what it's up to behind the scenes is the subject of much speculation, some of which isn't very reassuring. I bring this up because it reminds me that the yogis have long maintained our world is made of two basic kinds of matter, which are tangible (*sthula*) and subtle (*sukshma*) (usually *sthula* is translated as "gross" or "coarse," neither of which makes our physical body seem very appealing). The former is right at hand, we can see and touch it, taste it, play with it, make things out of it, and so on. The latter, though, is hidden from our everyday senses, we can't directly see and touch it (and by the way, I'm not suggesting an equivalence between the astronomer's so-called dark matter and the yogis' subtle, or that, as so many of our writers do, the yogis discovered things that modern science is only now catching up to). But it's not only the world that has a subtle dimension; each one of us supposedly does, too. It's technically known as the *sukshma sharira*, the "subtle body," which is criss-crossed by tens or even by some accounts hundreds of thousands of energy channels (*nadi*), and studded with energy centers called *cakras* ("wheels") and *marmans* ("joints").

We naturally tend to assume that the world accessible to our senses is the "real" world, and that the subtle is some kind of shadowy reflection. But the yogis say it's actually the other way around, since the subtle is the foundation for the tangible and so closer to the creator-source. How exactly we might access this world is difficult to fathom. Patanjali, in his usual succinct way, instructs us to direct the light of consciousness toward some object that will reveal things about that object that are subtle, concealed (*vyavahita*), and distant (*viprakrshta*) (YS 3.25). If we consult the commentators on this sutra to see if they can help figure out just what the master is talking about, we get the distinct impression that we have a better chance of wrapping our minds around dark matter than we have of penetrating the subtle.

This hasn't stopped our yoga teachers from avidly embracing this dimension, particularly the resident cakras. We have to admire their creativity and marketing skills, and their willingness to speak authoritatively about things they've probably never experienced directly. Go ahead and Google "cakra," and before you can say "muladhara," you're confronted—perhaps "assaulted" is a better word—with over two-and-a-half million hits. I've never quite understood what use we can make of that many possibilities. If I clicked on one every ten seconds and did nothing else but that, it would take me almost forty-eight years to get through them all.

Anyway, as we can see from this overload of evidence, modern teachers have taken the cakra ball and run with it, so to speak. They'll help you open your cakras, balance them, and heal them—though we know for sure from the old texts they're closed, it's not clear how they got unbalanced or ill—they offer cakra retreats, and if you're curious about the condition of your cakras, there are any number of tests you can take to help figure that out. You can even visit a website that, drawing on Ayurveda, a "5,000 year-old healing tradition from India" (there's that number again), will introduce to Mr. Chakra who'll help you use their product to spruce up your cakras and make them shine (we might think that since the subtle world of cakras is closely associated with the feminine power, that it would be more appropriate to call on Ms. Chakra for assistance).

I'm a bit reluctant, after what I just said about modern teachers and their relationship with the subtle, to contribute my secondhand knowledge to the pot. But the subtle world is a beautiful and mysterious place that we students should be familiar with. I encourage you, though, to first study the primary sources (however flawed the available modern translations are considered to be) such as the "Investigation of the Six Centers"

(*Shat Cakra Nirupana*), just to get the lay of the land as surveyed by the old yogis, before you dig into popular modern authors.

The following is just a brief visit to the traditional subtle world.

» *I read in a yoga book recently that another name for our spine is* Meru Danda. *Can you elaborate on that?*

> Ishvara says: In this body are Meru and seven islands with their rivers, oceans, and countries. There we find those who thirst (*trshya*) for liberation, those who have taken a vow of silence (*muni*), all the constellations and planets, sacred shrines, the Moon and Sun, and all of the creatures of the world.
>
> Freely adapted from *Shiva Samhita* 2.1–4

In order to answer this question, we need to first take a short trip to a very strange world—strange at least when compared to our familiar surroundings. For starters, this is not a place we can physically visit, like India or Disneyland, because it exists in the subtle realm accessible only to yogis in an intensely concentrated state of meditation. Of course, most of us haven't the wherewithal to actually undertake the journey to this subtle world, not yet at least, but fortunately we do have accounts generously provided us by a few psychonauts who made their way there and back again (though not all of them agree on the details of what they experienced). We're told that this world is an enormous disk supporting seven island continents, six of them arranged in neat concentric rings around a central "bull's-eye." Each continent (except the bull's-eye) is twice the size of the one it surrounds, and each is separated from its neighbors by an ocean, though only the innermost is salty like ours—the others are filled with sugarcane juice, wine, clarified butter or ghee, curds, cream, and milk (some reports describe the sixth sea as one of milk, and the outermost one of fresh water). All this is girdled by a mountain range estimated to be five hundred million *yojanas* in extent. (The exact length of a *yojana* is a subject of yet another debate among experts; some insist it's closer to five miles, others stretch it out to eight or nine. I'm certainly not qualified to settle this matter, so let's just say the world-circling mountain is at least two-and-a-half *billion* miles long, a little bit less than that of the distance from Earth to Neptune.) Last but not least, this whole magnificent construct perches on the head (or heads, sometimes seven in number, sometimes a thousand) of an immense serpent (who, in one yoga tradition, incarnated as Patanjali; see Chapter 4).

At the very hub of this world is an enormous golden mountain beside which the Himalayas would appear as mere speed bumps. In one account this mountain tops off at 84,000 *yojanas* (you can do the math), but height isn't the only thing about it that stands out (or up). This mountain is literally "turned on its head," since the diameter of its base is only half that of its summit, which gives it the appearance of the seed-cup of a lotus (according to one yogi at least; another maintains that the mountain is round like the morning sun, and burning with a smokeless flame). Four much smaller mountains buttress the golden mountain and keep it from tipping over, and each of these measures a mere ten thousand *yojanas* high, and is made of silver, emerald, crystal, and gold.

You might have already guessed that this immense golden mountain is popularly called Meru, though it's also known in some quarters as Good Meru (*sumeru*), Gold Mountain (*hemadri*), Jewel Peak (*ratna sanu*), Central Mountain (*karnikacala*), and God's Mountain (*deva parvata*). Scholars are uncertain about the origin of the name Meru, and some have tried to identify it with a real mountain, notably Tibet's Mount Kailasha, one of Shiva's favorite hangouts. But just as with the attempts to match the cakras to internal organs like the heart or brain, I'd take this with a grain or two of salt.

There's a good deal more we could say about Meru and the world that encircles it, but the information we have here will suffice for the question at hand. The essential thing to remember is that the mountain sits at the center of its world, like the hub of a wheel, so that everything in that world turns around it. It is symbolically seen as a link that joins the mundane world with the spiritual.

For the yogis then, our body is a microcosm, or "small world," which exists in a one-to-one equivalence with the macrocosm, or "great world." To paraphrase an old Western esoteric saying, "What's in here, in the body, is out there, in the world, and what's out there is in here. If it doesn't exist in here, it doesn't exist." Our spine, it should be obvious, is our "Mount Meru," and the main cakras strung along it are the seven islands. Our lives turn around our spine, not only physically and psychologically, but spiritually as well. That's because the spine houses our central energetic current, the *sushumna nadi*. This is the path taken by *kundalini* when, to fulfill our spiritual destiny, it climbs from the "base" of our mountain, physically located at the sacrum, to the summit at our crown and the heavenly "thousand-spoked" (*sahasrara*) center.

Now that's half the story. Where does *danda* come in? You may know of the Staff Pose (*dandasana*, see LoY 77). The staff is a second image used to characterize our spine and its role in our lives. The spine provides us with support, both in body and mind, as we go about our daily business, just as a wandering ascetic in India uses a staff to support himself in his endless peregrinations from one pilgrimage site to the next. What often isn't known is that *danda* also means "scepter." So not only does it represent the yogis' renunciant lives, but also the power and authority of the Self-realized being.

» *What are subtle channels* (nadis)?

The Sanskrit word *nadi* literally means "pipe" or "tube," though I prefer to render it as channel or current. The word refers both to physical nerves, veins, and arteries in the gross (*sthula*) body known to medical science, and to subtle (*sukshma*) channels in the subtle body through which the vital forces (*prana*), both positive and negative, circulate. John Woodroffe (1865–1936), a High Court judge in British India during the first two decades of the twentieth century, who wrote about Hindu Tantra under the pseudonym of Arthur Avalon, said of the nadis that "if they were revealed to the eye the body would present the appearance of a highly complicated chart of ocean currents. Superficially the water seems one and the same. But examination shows that it is moving with varying degrees of force in all directions."[5] In some texts, nadis are called *hitas* ("salutary," i.e., salutary rays) or *siras*.

The Hatha yogis believe that purity of the physical *and* subtle body is a necessary precondition for purity of mind. In the average person, the nadis are clogged, so the prana cannot flow freely through the body, leading to fatigue, disease, and decay. The Hatha yogis have various techniques to open the nadis, such as asana, pranayama, and the so-called six cleansings (*shat kriya*), which lead to a condition called the "purity of the channels" (*nadi shuddhi*). According to the *Hatha Yoga Pradipika* (2.19–20), when the nadis are purified, the yogi's body becomes light and perfectly healthy, she can hold her breath for a longer time, and the "fire in the belly" is stoked.

The number of nadis in the body is a matter of debate: various texts number them anywhere from 350,000 to 72,000 (e.g., HYP 1.39, 4.18). Of this last number Joseph Campbell writes that it's a "mythic magnitude, related to a science rather of a symbolic than of a strictly factual order";[6] in other words, we shouldn't take these numbers too literally, they simply indicate that there are countless nadis in the body. The entire network of nadis in the body is sometimes called the "wheel of channels" (*nadi cakra*).

The origin of the nadis is also disputed. In some texts, the nadis originate in the heart and stretch out, like the roots of a tree, in all directions. A few of the early Upanishads (e.g., BU 2.1.19; CU 8.6.6; KU 6.16; cf. *Prashna* 3.6), which number 101 nadis, follow this teaching. Other traditions originate the nadis in an egg-shaped "bulb" (*kanda*) located sometimes at the base of the spine (in the root *cakra*), sometimes in the middle of the body.

In keeping with the way the yogis typically deal with large numbers, the tens or hundreds of thousands of nadis are first whittled down to a far smaller number of significant nadis, usually fourteen, and then to the three most essential:

1. *Sushumna nadi* is the subtle central channel running through the spinal column from the opening in the kanda called the "Brahma gate" (*brahma dvara*) in the root cakra at the coccyx to the "Brahma fissure" (*brahma randhra*, the sutura frontalis in Western anatomy) or "Brahma cave" (*brahma bila*) at the crown. An old Tantric text, the *Investigation of the Six Centers* (*Shat Cakra Nirupana*), says that sushumna is "as subtle as a spider's thread . . . beautiful like a chain of

lightning . . . the awakener of pure knowledge; the embodiment of all Bliss" (v. 2).

2. The "comfort channel" (*ida nadi*, also called *shashi*, "Moon") is the "pale" left-hand channel, coiling around the central channel from the kanda to the left nostril. It represents the cooling, feminine energy of the body.

3. The "tawny channel" (*pingala nadi*, also called *mihira*, "Sun") is the "reddish" right-hand channel, coiling around the central channel from the kanda to the right nostril. It represents the body's heating, masculine energy.

As ida and pingala leave the kanda and spiral up around sushumna, they meet at five points along the way, each point marking the location of a cakra. Their sixth and final meeting comes at the place behind the mid-brow, at the "wheel of command" (*ajna cakra*), forming a knot called the "triple braid of release" (*mukta triveni*) or "triple peak" (*tri kuta*). From here, ida and pingala pass to the left and right nostrils, respectively, while the sushumna continues on to the crown of the head.

In the non-yogi, the entrance to sushumna at the base of the spine is blocked by the slumbering kundalini (see below). For such an individual, prana then is said to flow only through the ida and pingala nadis, and not through the sushumna. This condition represents "externalized" consciousness, that is, consciousness that is involved in the material world, supported by the alternating positive and negative currents of the body. As the *Hatha Yoga Pradipika* says, prana flowing in the ida and pingala is the cause of "day and night," that is, time (*kala*) and death.

In general, yogic techniques such as asana and pranayama are designed to devitalize the ida and pingala nadis by withdrawing their supply of prana and directing it to the brahma dvara. This concentration of energy in the root cakra creates an enormous heat, which jolts the kundalini awake as if a snake were whacked by a stick (HYP 3.66). Aroused, the kundalini then blasts off through the central channel to the crown. This results in samadhi, which is said to swallow (HYP 4.17) time and death, in other words, to lead to immortality and Self-liberation.

» *What are the cakras?*

A cakra is literally a "wheel" or "circle" (cakras are also known and pictured as "lotuses," *padmas*). It's generally reported that there are six or seven of them located along the central channel (*sushumna nadi*) in the subtle body, but that's just one particular model; other models include eight, nine, or twelve or more cakras. These numbers, however, are dwarfed by those noted in some sources, which number the cakras well into the tens of thousands; however, as with all yoga numbers of this magnitude, they're not to be taken literally, they're only meant to indicate that there are "lots and lots" of them.

The six main cakras, or wheels, along the sushumna can be visualized in different ways. For me they're "signposts" along a path from the depths of our unconscious mind to the heights of super-consciousness. The lower wheels pertain to more mundane feelings of physical embodiment and sexuality; the higher ones become increasingly "spiritual," leading from altruism to insight to ultimate transcendence (in some descriptions the *sahasrara*, the crown center, is situated *above* the crown, out of the body, providing an apt image for transcendence). As I understand the cakra system, the cakras are for the average person either unrealized or only realized in the "lower" realms of physical embodiment, sexuality, and self-survival, while the "higher" emotions remain still unrealized.

The idea behind the practice of Hatha Yoga then is to open these centers of consciousness by first awakening the dormant spiritual energy (*kundalini*) in the "root-support" (*muladhara*) center at the base of the spine, then driving this energy up through the central subtle channel to its spiritual fulfillment in the crown. The old texts describe a variety of methods to accomplish this awakening, mostly pranayama and mudra (see below). We are, however, frequently warned that attempting this movement of spiritual energy without expert guidance can be dangerous, since if the physical body is unprepared, the enormous charge of spiritual energy can blow the circuits of our nervous system.

There has been a steady stream of articles in popular yoga literature, not to mention DVDs and workshops, that make use of the cakras in very imaginative ways. As I mentioned earlier, the cakras are typically depicted in stripped-down versions, which may make them more accessible to a general audience but at the same time lessens their power as transformative agents.

Traditionally each cakra includes a "seed" (*bija*) mantra (i.e., a nasalized Sanskrit consonant such as *LAM* or *RAM*), which aids meditation on that center; a geometric shape (e.g., a square or crescent moon); a traditional element (e.g., earth or water); a totem animal (e.g., an elephant or crocodile), which represents particular qualities of that center; and tutelary deities, each holding multiple symbolic objects (e.g., the *vajra* or thunderbolt). All of these are surrounded by a certain number of "petals" or "spokes," each one signified by one of fifty *nagari* vowels or consonants.

>> *I'm interested in the cakras, and as I read about them in the old books, every now and then there's a reference to the "knots." What exactly are these knots and how does the yogi deal with them?*

When the knots are all cut
that bind one's heart on earth;
Then a mortal becomes immortal. . . .

Chandogya Upanishad 6.15 (translation by Patrick Olivelle)

This Kumbhaka called Bhastrika should be specially practiced, as it enables [the breath] to break through the three knots that are firmly placed in the Sushumna.

Hatha Yoga Pradipika 2.67

Apparently it's not challenging enough to first purify the physical body, then the subtle energy channels, then get a handle on the pranic energy, charge it and direct to the base cakra (*muladhara*), wake the "sleeping serpent" (*kundalini*), and finally move that energy up through the central channel (*sushumna*) to its terminus at the crown center. No, it seems there are obstacles along the course of the sushumna, called "knots" (*granthi*), which must be pierced before the whole process can be completed.

As evidenced by the passage above from *Chandogya Upanishad* (which dates to at least to 600 B.C.E.), the earliest accounts of the granthis referred to an indeterminate number of knots, all located in the heart, which were created there by "lurking" (*shrita*) desires (CU 6.14). These knots were said to keep the yogi tied to the mundane world and prevent him from reaching the divine.

By the time of the *Hatha Yoga Pradipika* (about two thousand years later) the knots had been reduced to three, distributed among three cakras, which differ from text to text. But regardless of their location, the three knots always have the same hierarchical arrangement: the lowest knot is Brahma, the middle is Vishnu, and the uppermost is called Rudra (an older name for Shiva).

As you can see from the *Hatha Yoga Pradipika* quote above, Svatmarama instructs us to pierce the knots through the practice of the Bellows (*bhastrika*), a traditional pranayama. My own feeling about this practice is that it's best learned from an experienced teacher. If improperly performed, Bellows can lead to headaches or stir up deep-seated emotional issues that we may not have the experience to properly self-treat. So I won't say anything more about this practice here. In any case, it's not clear to me if the practice of bhastrika pierces the knots to clear the path for kundalini, or if the practice works instead to stimulate the kundalini, who will then do the piercing herself as she rises through the central channel.

I found one teacher who has a slightly different understanding of the function of the knots. Yogi Hari sees the knots as "safety valves," that "God has created so that this Divine energy would not be prematurely awakened and create a short circuit within you." This seems like an eminently logical way to look at the knots. He goes on to say that such knots are "inherent in every atom of creation. Without them, we would be having atomic explosions all the time. This planet would be the sun again."[7]

» I've heard so much about kundalini. Could you talk a little about it?

Well, I can talk about *her*, sure. In the West, we typically think of masculine energy as active and creative, and feminine energy as passive and receptive; but in India, these roles are often reversed so that it's the feminine "power," *Shakti* (from the verb *shak,* "to be strong or powerful"), that begets, nourishes, and finally reabsorbs the world and all its creatures at the end of its life cycle. Her world-play (*lila*) is silently witnessed by her spouse, masculine *Shiva,* the "auspicious one," who's forever unmoving and unmoved. It's important to remember that while we might talk about Shakti and Shiva as separate figures, they can't really be divorced; ultimately they're nothing other than the positive and negative "poles" of the foundation of all creation, Brahman, the "vast abyss."

After she has playfully created the world and each individual, Shakti divides: half of her remains active as the life force, *prana,* that pervades and sustains the universe; her other half comes to rest and slumbers in each of us, it's said, in a secret cave at the base of our spine. Although she's known by many names, most of them expressing her spring-like coiled shape, Shakti is most popularly pictured as a goddess-serpent wound three-and-a-half (though sometimes eight) times around herself, and so is called *Kundalini,* or "Coiled One." The seventeenth-century *Investigation of the Six Centers* (v. 11) declares:

> Her sweet murmur is like the . . . hum of swarms of love-mad bees. . . . It is She who maintains all the beings of the world . . . and shines in the cavity of the root . . . like a chain of brilliant lights.

Carl Jung writes that the symbol of the serpent represents "the hidden or underground divinity concealed in the recesses of physical nature and in the instinctual forces of the human psyche itself."[8] She is the common denominator, the bridge between the seemingly separate individuals of this world, the Mother of us all. She, too, is the source of the collective unconscious and the eternal images (archetypes) through which all the people of the world express their deepest longings and insights.

For hundreds of years in India, the mythic elements of her story have served as fertile ground for intense devotion and meditation as a path to Self-realization. Kundalini is a symbol of the infinite spiritual potency, coiled like a spring ready to unleash its energy, residing in each of us at the subtle root of our being. Snakes have long represented both knowledge and, since they periodically slough their skins, self-transformation. But Kundalini's hibernation reminds us that we are "asleep" to our own authentic identity. It's said that her mouth covers the entrance to the *sushumna nadi*, our path to liberation. For those devoted to awakening kundalini, the true aim of our practice is to bestir ourselves from our spiritual dormancy and move toward full self-realization.

The origin of Hatha Yoga (Version 2)

So they took up Jonah and cast him forth into the sea. . . . Now the Lord had prepared a great fish to swallow up Jonah. And Jonah was in the belly of the fish three days and three nights.

JONAH, 1:15–17

Once upon a time there was a fisherman who was pulled overboard into the sea. Alternately, once upon another time there was a poor child, born under unlucky stars and planets, who was tossed into the sea. In any case, however he got there, the drowning fisherman/child was swallowed by a huge fish, usually described as a whale (though of course a whale isn't a fish). Stuck inside the fish's belly, the fisherman/child was transported either to the sacred Moon Island or the bottom of the sea. Coincidentally (or maybe not) Shiva and Shakti also happened to be there; they'd sought a quiet place far from prying ears so that Shiva could instruct his wife in the secrets of yoga. But they didn't get far enough away, and while Shakti fell asleep during her husband's peroration, the fisherman/child took it all in. Shiva, suspecting that Shakti wasn't paying the closest attention, asked her: "Are you listening?" The fisherman/child, who was indeed listening very carefully, replied without thinking, "Yes!" Shiva was surprised to discover he'd been overheard but pleased nonetheless with the studious attention of the fisherman/child, and he initiated him into the secrets of his teaching, giving him the name Matsyendra, the "Lord of the Fish." Matsyendra then either emerged immediately from the fish's belly or decided to stay put and, after twelve years of refining his practice, was freed by a fisherman who caught the great fish and cut open its belly.

>> *Most students nowadays go to a yoga class or two a week, and maybe do a little home practice, but not much more than that. I've heard you say that in the old days, the yogis lived their practice. What was a yogi's daily practice like back then?*

Between all of our home and workplace responsibilities, between the kids and the spouse (or partner or parents), our friends, the boss and co-workers, and of course the dog, we often find it hard to free up the time during our busy day (or week or month) to maintain even a semblance of a personal yoga (asana) practice. You might be encouraged or challenged (but not disheartened, I hope) to know the daily schedule for a traditional Hatha Yoga practice. It's drawn from Brahmananda's *Moonlight* (*Jyotsna*, 2.48), a late-nineteenth-century commentary on the *Hatha Yoga Pradipika*.

MORNING: PRELIMINARY

The yogi wakes up at "dawn time" (*usha kala*), somewhere between 4:00 and 6:00 A.M. He immediately remembers his guru "in his head" (i.e., mind) and his chosen deity (*sveshta deva*, a deity "dear to oneself") "in his heart." Then he washes himself, brushes his teeth, and smears his body with holy ashes (*bhasman*, see below).

After this he performs a rite that's obligatory for all men of the upper three castes (who are called *dvija*, "twice-born"), a rite that's known as "junction" or "boundary" (*sandhya*), which he'll repeat at noon and twilight. As the name suggests, this rite is synchronized with daily changes in the light, the sacred "junctions" of sunrise, noon, and sunset (the four practices, described next, are also repeated at these junctions, with the fourth coming at midnight). The sandhya rite consists mainly of reciting what's probably the most well-known of all the Sanskrit mantras, the *gayatri* (a verse meter of twenty-four syllables): "Let us contemplate that beautiful splendor of the divine Savitri [solar god], that he may inspire our visions" (translation by Georg Feuerstein). These words are usually prefixed with *om* and what's called the "great utterance" (*maha vyahriti*), the words for the three worlds of "earth" (*bhur*), "mid-region" (*bhuvar*), and "heaven" (*svar*).

Now the yogi lays out his mat (Brahmananda recommends deer skin, but see below) and petitions in various ways for success in his practice of asanas. First he prostrates himself to Shiva and makes a firm resolution that "I shall practice asanas and pranayama to reach the goal of samadhi," then he salutes the "Infinite" (*ananta*), who is lord of the snakes (*nagas*, whose name is also *shesha*, "Remainder"). Now he conducts his asana practice, finishing with Corpse (*shava*) if he is tired, but if he isn't tired, then Corpse isn't needed.

To get ready for pranayama and retention (*kumbhaka*), the yogi practices Inverted Action [Seal] (*viparita karani mudra*) (nowadays called Shoulder Stand). This will prepare the body for the "throat bond" (*jalandhara bandha*, literally "net-holding bond"), which is needed for retention.

Next comes pranayama. The yogi sits in the Adept's Pose (*siddha*) with a focused mind, and on the first day performs ten rounds of pranayama, increasing the number of rounds by five for each succeeding day until reaching eighty rounds, which will take two weeks (it isn't clear from the text if the yogi should practice eighty rounds for each of the six pranayamas listed below, or for just one. I suspect that would be just one, since 240 rounds might take up to two hours). The formal practice begins with Moon-Sun (*candra surya*) breath, also known as With-the-Grain-Against-the-Grain (*viloma-anuloma*). Next come the Sun Piercing (*surya bhedana*) and Conqueror (*ujjayi*) breaths, finishing up with "Make [the sound of] 'seet'" (*sitkari*) and/or Cooling (*shitali*) breaths, and finally Bellows (*bhastrika*). He may now stop or continue to do more pranayama.

After pranayama, the yogi sits in Lotus (*padma*) and practices reflection on the "subtle sound" in his right ear (*nada yoga*). This practice is described in detail in the fourth chapter of the *Hatha Yoga Pradipika* (briefly at 4.67–68, and more extensively at 4.80–102). Svatmarama instructs the yogi to sit in Liberated (*mukta*), use his hands to block or almost block the ears, eyes, nostrils, and mouth (though he also says to perform Shiva's Seal, *shambhavi mudra,* which means the eyes should be partially open), and listen with a focused mind for a sound in the right ear.

It is interesting to note that in the practices of asana and nada described in the *Hatha Yoga Pradipika*, the asanas are described over the course of about thirty-six verses, while the nada instruction takes up about forty verses. This shows us that 550 years ago, though it was just beginning to emerge as a practice that included more than just sitting poses, asana still took a backseat to breathing and meditation. Today, by contrast, asana is firmly in the driver's seat, and breathing and meditation aren't even in the car—they're lonely hitchhikers beside the road.

The yogi is reminded that all these practices should be done as an offering to the deity. To finish the morning practice, he takes a hot water bath, then completes his "daily duties."

Noon

The noon practice is the same as the morning practice. After practicing, the yogi has lunch, but is cautioned to eat only food that's wholesome and recommended for yogis. His diet is prescribed at *Hatha Yoga Pradipika* 1.58–63 (and compare GS 5.16–29). Among forbidden things are foods that are bitter, salty, spicy, hot, or stale; meat; and reheated foods (no leftovers). Among the recommended foods are grains, some dairy products, sweets, and water. To help digestion, I suppose, he finishes his meal with some cardamom or clove or, if he prefers, camphor and betel leaf.

Afternoon

The afternoon is spent either (1) studying the "liberation texts" (*mokshashashtra*), such as the *Bhagavad Gita* or the Vedic Upanishads; (2) listening to the "old tales," the Puranas; or (3) devotedly reciting the deity's name.

Evening

The yogi repeats most of the afternoon practice beginning exactly seventy-two minutes (three *ghatika*; one ghatika is twenty-four minutes) before sundown (he's advised not to do Inverted Action here or at midnight). Afterward he eats his evening meal.

Midnight

The yogi repeats the evening practice (GS at 5.89 recommends a fifth practice, in which case the start times would have to be adjusted to accommodate a practice about every four and a half to five hours).

As we can see, being a yogi was once a full-time job, or better yet, a life's occupation. It's hard to say exactly how time-consuming each of the four (or five) practices was, but by a conservative estimate surely each lasted around ninety minutes, which means the yogi devoted a minimum of six hours a day to practice, not counting his afternoon study session, which might have lasted another hour.

» What did the old yogis use for a mat?

The yogi should establish a "stable seat for himself in a pure place . . . [with] a cloth, deerskin, or *kusha*-grass for covering."

Bhagavad Gita 6.11

Nowadays we generally practice indoors on a sticky mat to keep ourselves from sliding on the bare floor or carpet. In the early 1980s, the typical mat (usually green in color) had a very short life span of a few months. Depending on the frequency and style of your practice, it would soon start to shed little bits of green dandruff all over the floor. But the mats were fairly inexpensive, especially if you bought a big roll of material and cut your own to size. Over the last several years, the quality of mats, and consequently their price, has changed dramatically. A mat can now cost upwards of a hundred dollars, and is usually made of some kind of heavy, indestructible rubber-like material that, no matter how often and how hard we practice on it, will surely outlast us and likely become family heirlooms.

In the old, old days, the preferred "sticky mat" was either a tiger skin or a deerskin. In the tenth-century *Flood of Kula Treatise* (*Kula Arnava Tantra*, 15.32–33), we find an extensive list of materials and their benefits or drawbacks. "The wise shall reject the seat made of bamboo, stone, earth, wood, grass or sprout; such seats only bring poverty, disease and misery. A seat made of cotton, wool, cloth, skin of lion, tiger or deer brings good fortune."

Some of the material recommendations, and their supposed benefits, are more than a little strange. A tiger skin leads to success in all things and is a good seat covering for salvation while a deerskin brings knowledge, presumably of the spiritual kind (the tiger and the deer, however, may have a different perspective on salvation and knowledge). Various cloths, as in the *Flood* treatise, also have beneficial results: in general cotton is good for curing disease, while silk insures success in rites promoting welfare and the fulfillment of all desires. Some texts warn that seats of stone and wood bring poverty; others say exactly the opposite, that they will bring wealth. (Which is true, I can't say. I suppose the best thing to do is try each out for a time while closely monitoring the fluctuations of your bank account.) Cane, which might be the "bamboo" mentioned in the *Flood*, is also given positive reviews in some texts. It's supposed to increase love, though of whom or what isn't specified, so I'd be a bit cautious with this material.

Do you want to bewitch someone or counteract poison? Then you'll need to sit on a sheepskin. Do you want someone to hate you? It's not clear exactly why someone would desire this, but if you do, you'll need the skin of a dog (beware the ire of the ASPCA if you're discovered skinning Fido). How about something a little more diabolical, like paralyzing or ruining an enemy? You'll need a cowhide for the former, a horsehide for the latter. Or maybe you'd prefer to cut to the chase and kill someone outright? For this you'll need the skin of a buffalo.

I assume here we're dealing with a bit of exaggeration in all of these suggestions, and I'm absolutely *not* advocating the use of animal hides to settle unresolved conflicts with co-workers or family members. But Para-mahamsa Yogananda, author of the widely read *Autobiography of a Yogi*, was apparently quite serious about the benefits of tiger and deer hides. According to him, when the meditating yogi tries to withdraw his senses from involvement with the outside world and aim them inward toward the Self, an uninsulated body-mind will be pulled this way and that, and surely perturbed, by the "upward flow" of the life force and the contrary "downward pull of the earth currents."[9] It would seem we're still subject to the same energetic turbulence that bothered our yogic forebears. When seated on tiger or deer hide, however, the yogi is fully protected from the tug-of-war between his prana and the planet. Fortunately, Yogananda allows that animal hides aren't necessary in the modern world (though he doesn't say why exactly). We may instead sit on a woolen blanket covered with silk, which apparently repels certain earth currents better than does cotton, certainly welcome news to the endangered tigers of the world, not to mention the other animals on the yogis' hit list.

» *According to tradition, what's the best time of day to practice?*

Just as for a yogi's orientation in space—always to the east or north—and his choice of seat materials, it should come as no surprise that the times prescribed for practice are carefully regulated. As the holy days for many faiths tend to be clustered around significant changes in the yearly light, especially the equinoxes and solstices—as with the Christian Easter and Jewish Passover—similarly, yogis are enjoined to practice at significant sacred "junctions" (*sandhya*) in the daily alterations of light and dark, such as sunrise, noon, sunset, or midnight.

The *Gheranda Samhita* (5.88–89) offers options for three different practice schedules: three times daily, with practice occurring every eight hours (at sunrise, noon, and sunset); or five times daily or eight times daily, every three hours.

A thrice-a-day routine goes all the way back to Vedic times, and is still followed today by pious Hindus. The contents of the ceremony varies somewhat depending on the chosen deity and affiliation of the worshiper, but in general it's packed with benedictory mantras, pranayama, and meditation. A much later and simpler sandhya is outlined in the fourteenth-century *Brihad Yogi Yajnavalkya Smrti,* stripped down to virtual bathing, mantra recitation, and meditation. Every twice-born Hindu (*dvija,* referring to the three upper castes; the lowest caste *shudras* were forbidden to participate) is enjoined to unfailingly honor these junctions with a number of potent, Brahman-created mantras. The goal apparently is twofold: to protect the laws that keep the universe running smoothly and to expiate personal transgressions. Anyone who dodges this duty is in for some big trouble: he'll be demoted to the lowest caste, then reborn into his next life as a dog. Woof!

I hazard to guess that there are very few of us nowadays with the time or inclination to perform eight, five, or even three daily practices—no matter what future canine life we are threatened with. So if we must limit ourselves to a single daily session, it's usually recommended it be conducted either at sunrise or sunset. It's believed that during these junctions, the balance between the waxing or waning light and the waning or waxing dark has a soothing effect on our own internal, often-conflicted forces of light and dark, and makes for a harmonious practice.

» *Is there a particular way I should face when I practice?*

The east, indeed, is the region of the gods, for this reason he (the sacrificer) looks toward the East.

Brahmana of the Hundred Paths (*Shatapatha Brahmana*),
1.9.3.13, ca. 700 B.C.E.

Space, writes Alain Danielou, is the "substratum of the cosmos . . . the abode, the source, of all forms." The cardinal and ordinal directions then, "the determinants of space, have a special significance," which reveal and express "particular powers." This means that our orientation in space is an "essential element"[10] of all rituals, including yoga practice. Several of the old yoga books (such as the YY 5.14, VS 2.6, and GS 5.48) advise us to face either east (*pranmukha*) or north (*udanmukha*) when practicing.

East is the quarter of the rising Sun, a symbol of the dawn of spiritual "illumination" or insight, which we hope to realize through our practice. North is the quarter of the North or Pole Star, called *dhruva,* "fixed, firm, eternal," and *grahadhara,* the "pivot of the planets," because it's believed the planets and other stars are tied to it by invisible cords, and so attached seem to turn about it. The North Star then is a symbol of the "fixed, firm, eternal" Self. By facing toward its quarter, we acknowledge that the Self is the "pivot" not only of our practice, but our lives as well.

There seems to be one more down-to-earth reason for facing east or north. Rudra Shivananda, a retired Silicon Valley "technology professional" who has now dedicated his life to the "well-being of humanity,"[11] bases his recommendations for spatial orientation not on the stars but on the west-to-east axial rotation of the Earth (which of course gives the illusion that the Sun "rises" in the east and "sets" in the west). Ideally, he says, we should face east when practicing because that's the way the Earth is turning. He claims that facing west is something like facing against a train's direction of motion, which is upsetting to many people.

So a western-facing practice could cause a kind of "yoga nausea." But if we can't face east, he continues (and its difficult to imagine a situation where our access to facing east is blocked), then we should align ourselves with the Earth's magnetic field and face north.

» What is "placing" (nyasa)?

The yogi should sit on his platform and take Lotus Pose. Next, as advised by his guru, he should place (*nyasa*) his guru and the gods in various areas of his body, then purify his nadis to ready himself for pranayama.

Gheranda Samhita 5.38

Thus propounding to me in order the mystical sanctification (*nyasa*) of the limbs, sage, meter, deity and their application forming the sheath of Brahma and the encased nectar—the universal soul himself became merged in yoga.

Vasishtha Samhita 6.24

I imagine that most Westerners are familiar with (if not regular performers of) the sign of the cross, most closely associated with the Roman Catholic Church. The worshiper traces with her right hand the shape of a cross with points on her head, heart, and shoulders, demonstrating her belief in the redemptive power of the Christian crucifixion; at the same time, she recites mentally or aloud what's called the Trinitarian formula, words that summon the members of the Trinity, the Father, Son, and Holy Spirit.

Similar ritual elements make up a yoga exercise known as "placing" or "fixing" (*nyasa*, from the verb *as*, "to lay or put upon"), traditionally performed as a preparation for practice or worship. The yogi mindfully touches a prescribed body part (usually with the right hand), and charges it with an accompanying mantra, which may be a seemingly nonsense syllable, a *nagari* vowel or consonant (for more on *nagari*, see Chapter 2), each here called a "mother" (*matrika*) because of its supposed creative potency, or given the name of a god or goddess. *The Daily Practice of the Hindus* summarizes the idea behind "placing" thusly:

Before entering into the worship of God, the whole body with its various organs, must be dedicated to God, Who should be considered as dwelling in every part of it. As a temple is consecrated before it becomes a sacred place of worship, so before God is invoked, this body (the true temple of God) should be dedicated to him [and I might add here, "or her"].[12]

There are numerous variations of placing. Some are short and sweet, involving no more that a simple touch of a single body part, such as the heart, infused with a brief mantra, such as so'ham, "I am He," or sa'ham, "I am She." Alternatively, the placing can be very complicated and time consuming. The *matrika nyasa,* for example, requires two installations of the fifty "mothers," the characters of the *nagari* alpha-syllabary believed to embody the different parts and limbs of the body of the Goddess. This is done first internally in the cakras, and again a second time externally in a laundry list of spots from head to feet (including the teeth and oral cavity). The essential principle behind all forms of placing, writes John Woodroffe, is the conviction that transformation of the way we think about ourselves results ultimately in the transformation of our being.

Rather than try to describe in detail the many placings I ran across in my research, which would take up far too much space, I'll give you an example of placing taken from the above quoted *Daily Practice.* The practice is called *kha sparsha,* which means something like "touching the centers (*kha*) of the body." There are usually twelve centers that are touched in sequence, but we'll skip the ascetic's "tuft" at the top of the head, since I assume there are few people reading this book living a spartan, self-denying lifestyle.

Traditionally the placing is done with the middle and ring fingers of the right hand. I like to repeat the mantra silently to myself rather than saying it aloud. Somewhere I once heard that a whispered mantra is one hundred times more effective than a spoken mantra, and a mantra recited silently (e.g., mentally) to oneself is one hundred times more effective than a whispered one. (Alas, I don't remember the source for this suggestion, but based on my firm belief in this practice it must have been pretty authoritative.)

I won't here go into all the prejudices against the left hand; they're just as powerful in India as they are in the West. The Sanskrit word for "right" is *dakshina*, "sincere, pleasing," while "left" is *vama*, "adverse, unfavorable; cruel, wicked." (If you're left-handed, please note I'm quoting from a dictionary, and not making this stuff up.) I encourage my left-handed students to ignore these outdated superstitions and freely use their dominant hand for the practice of placing.

How you use this practice will be determined by your goal. If you just want to enliven your body in preparation for an asana practice, then a firm touch will suffice. Perhaps instead you want to meditate on a particular quality, like compassion or courage, or your favorite deity. Then your touch might infuse some particular thought or energetic quality.

A quick Sanskrit review to help with pronunciation. Seven of the eleven mantras end with a *visarga* (see Chapter 1). You may recall that the visarga is transliterated as an under-dotted *h*, which indicates that the previous vowel should be echoed. For example, *manah* is pronounced ma-nuh-huh. Below you'll find a pronunciation guide for all the mantras in the sequence.

When there are two things to touch—eyes, ears, etc.—we're supposed to touch the right one first; again, I give you my permission to touch the left first if the left side is your dominant side.

MANTRA	SAY	ENGLISH	TOUCH
vak	vahk	speech	lips
manah	ma-nuh-huh	mind	lower lip
pranah	pra-nuh-huh	breath	nostrils
cakshuh	chak-shu-huh	eyes	eyes
shrotam	shro-tum	ears	ears
nabih	na-be-he	navel	navel
hridayam	hri-di-um	heart	heart
kantah	kan-tuh-huh	throat	throat
sirahah	sheer-uh-huh	head	head
bahu	bah-hu	hands	hands

With this last mantra, cross one hand to the opposite shoulder, then the other hand to the other shoulder, and say, *Om yasho balam astu*, "let there be honor (*yazas*) and strength (*bala*)." Finally bring your hands together in front of your sternum in *anjali mudra* (see below).[13]

>> *Every time I see a picture of a practicing yogi, I have to wonder what all that paraphernalia he's wearing and holding is for and what it means. Can you explain anything about this?*

The old yogis did a lot of wandering and so traveled extremely lightly, carrying only those things needed to maintain a very basic existence. Let's start with the first part of your question, what does a yogi wear? Are you asking this because you want to dress like a yogi? Well, if you were to "dress" like some of them, you'd attract a lot of attention. I'm referring to the yogis who traditionally wander about in their birthday suits, covered only by a nice thick coating of ashes (see below). A yogi who chooses this particular style of non-dress, likely in honor of the lord of yoga, Shiva, is said to be *digambara*, "clothed in the sky," which is also one of Shiva's many nicknames. With his nakedness the yogi is telling the world that he's left behind *all* worldly attachments, including that of sexuality. But not all yogis go naked. Some wear a skimpy loin cloth (*langoti*) about their waist, from which hangs a narrow strip of cloth (*kaupina*) to hide the privates, and some dress in a full robe, traditionally yellow or saffron-orange. We might also look for a sacred thread (*janeo*), presented to the yogi on his coming-of-age ceremony.

Now, what does a yogi tote around? He usually has a staff, which may be decorated in various ways; for example, the staff may be topped with a skull (if we can call that a "decoration"). From a practical point of view, the staff serves a dual purpose, offering both support and self-protection in the yogi's wanderings, "but in a religious and mystical context it is the pastoral staff, the rod of divination, the magic wand, and thus a symbol of spiritual power."[14]

Instead of a staff, the yogi might carry a trident (*trishula*), which not only serves the two aforementioned practical purposes—and is certainly a more formidable weapon than a staff—but also once again honors Shiva, its most famous wielder. The three prongs, moreover, represent, among other things, the three "strands" (*guna,* see Chapter 4) or qualities of nature, a reminder that Shiva (at least according to his devotees) is the force that creates, preserves, and then recycles the universe. Along with a staff the yogi may carry an assortment of other items: a small crutch (*acal*), which he uses to support an arm or chin during meditation; a fan made of peacock feathers or animal hair, to drive off evil spirits; a water pot (*kamendalu*), which is also a symbol of his ascetic life; and a begging bowl (*kharpara* "skull"), which may be a coconut shell, a gourd, or an actual human skull.

A yogi also won't go anywhere without his rosary (*mala*), which is typically made from what are called "Rudra-eyed" (*rudraksha*) berries. These represent Shiva's "third eye," and each has a number of sides or "faces," anywhere from one to eleven. The most common number is five, which represents Shiva's five faces. The rarest number is one, supposedly possessed only by kings. If you find a one-face berry, be sure to hang onto it, for it guarantees a life of power, wealth, and joy. Eleven seems to be the most auspicious number, but these berries, called "non-spilled" (*askanda*), are worn only by celibates.

THE "FIVE FACES" OF SHIVA

Since Shiva is the ruler of all space, he needs to keep a sharp eye on all four major directions, as well as what's going on above him. Thus he has five faces. Each has its own personality—north, east, and west seem pleasant enough, but the southern face, we're warned, is best avoided. Each face is connected with one of the five traditional elements (earth, water, fire, air, and ether), one of the five senses (for Shiva also rules over them), and a physical organ. For each of the five directions, Shiva carries symbolic objects—weapons like spears and hatchets seem to be quite popular—and makes a symbolic gesture with his (many) hands.

» Traditionally, where did yogis live?

The yogi shouldn't start his practice in a distant place where there's no security, or in a forest where there's no food, or in a crowd where there's much distraction. If he does he won't succeed. Instead he should live in a peaceful, law-abiding country, where there are plenty of alms available.

Freely adapted from *Gheranda Samhita* 5.2–5

The cartoon shows a solitary yogi sitting atop a mountain. Just below him, clinging precariously to the steep mountainside, is a man who has struggled his way to the summit to ask the wise one to reveal to him the meaning of life. "Google it," says the yogi.

In the West we have a popular image of the yogi living as a hermit far from the madding crowd in a cave on some lofty, isolated Himalayan peak. It's a romantic image, but ask yourself: could a yogi find enough food and water and wood for a fire up there on top of Old Smokey while also presumably spending most of his day in practice and study? It's highly unlikely, though we can't completely discount the possibility.

In fact the old Hatha Yoga books specifically instruct the yogi not to reside in distant places, but in a *sudesha dharmika,* a "good, righteous country" (GS 5.5) where food is good and abundant (*subhiksha*) (HYP 1.12), and which is ruled by a righteous king and populated by similarly high-minded subjects. He's further cautioned to live neither too close to town, which could be a distraction to his practice, nor too far away, since he'll need to visit there each day to depend on the kindness of strangers and beg for his daily bread.

Now what about the yogi's suburban domicile itself? He's directed to build a one-room, windowless hut, called either a *matha* (in the HYP, SS, and YY) or a *kutira* (in the GS), though both words mean about the same thing, "hut" or "cottage." The interior should be clean and bug free, "perfumed with the smoke of frankincense" (*Yoga Tattva Upanishad* 33), its walls washed with lime or, more commonly, smeared with cow dung. This last decor advice may give us pause, but research reveals that cow dung is a natural insulator, that it binds mud bricks and prevents them from falling apart, and that spread on a dirt floor it readily absorbs any spilled liquid. The surrounding yard should be enclosed by a low wall, have a well for water and a raised, canopied platform (*mandapa*) for the yogi's daily practice, which, considering the size of the hut, is done mostly outdoors.

Svatmarama uses the *matha* as a metaphor for Hatha Yoga itself. "For those who are suffering from all kinds of pain," he writes, "Hatha Yoga is like a *matha* which gives us refuge" (*samashraya*, HYP 1.10).

» *Why did some yogis cover themselves with ashes?*

Yogis believe that by burning something to ashes, we can liberate and purify its essence, which still has traces of the original cosmic matter. Ashes then are powerful stuff, "food" from the god of fire, especially those ashes that come from sacrificial or cremation fires. For us these signify death, but for the yogi who covers himself in such ashes, he's announcing that he's "burned his bridges" with the mundane world, sacrificed his karma in the "fire" of austerity (*tapas*), and is now (or at least wishes he was) immortal.

The first ash smearer was Shiva. It's said he once incinerated the entire universe, including his buddy deities, Brahma and Vishnu, with a yogic phaser beam from his "third eye," then rubbed the ashes on his body.

Ashes are called *bhasman*, which literally means "devouring"—that is, what is left after a fire "devours" the material being burned. When you're smeared with ashes, you're said to be *vibhuti*, which also means "mighty, powerful." Practically, it's claimed that a coat of ashes protects the yogi's naked body on the cooler days of winter in India.

» *I've always wondered where the asanas come from. Any ideas about that?*

Yes, I do indeed have ideas, but whether or not they're the right ideas, I have no idea.

One possible origin of some of the asanas is suggested by Vyasa's commentary on *Yoga Sutra* 2.46. This is the sutra that sets the standard for a successful asana in Patanjali's opinion, that is, "steady and comfortable." You may remember that Patanjali doesn't actually name any asanas, but Vyasa in his commentary names a handful, for example, Hero and Staff. Then he writes, "The Curlew (*kraunca*) and the other seats may be understood by actually seeing a curlew and the other animals seated." This suggests to me that Vyasa is saying that some asanas are imitations of the "seats," or typical poses, of certain animals. If we look in the *Gheranda Samhita* (2.3–6), we find that half of the thirty-two asanas listed either are named after or have names in some way related to an animal; for example, there's Lion, Fish, Peacock, Rooster, Tortoise, Bull, Frog, Camel, Serpent, and Locust.

Another possibility is that asanas could simply be formalizations of natural human postures. In a 1957 *Scientific American* article, author Gordon Hewes includes fifty line drawings of different human postures, from photos taken all over the world. The majority of the figures are kneeling, squatting, or seated on the ground, and most of the postures could be found in one form or another in the *Encyclopedia of Traditional Asanas* (2006). Four drawings show figures standing on one leg in positions very similar to Tree (*vṛksha*), and six others show figures sitting on a flat surface like a bench, which resemble several seated asanas described in the *Encyclopedia*.

Yet another possibility is that the asanas derived from other disciplines. There's little doubt that many postures we know today were borrowed from twentieth-century body disciplines like Western gymnastics and Indian wrestling. For example, the pose named Hanuman is obviously the deep splits in Western gymnastics; I'm told that the pose named Swinging (*lola*) is an arm strengthener that comes from Indian wrestling, where it is also called Swinging, or *jhula* in Hindi.

My good friend Stu Sovatsky believes that many of the asanas are what he calls "apollonian formulations"—or, in plain English, static representations of (ready?) "dionysian," or spontaneous expressions of "yearning, quaking, shaking, davening [or shuckling], throbbing, swaying, and bodily tumescences." Stu suggests that originally asanas were impelled by a "force, a divine *shakti*" that inspired the yogi to "worshipfully stretch and develop her own body, beyond her own will's choices and dictates." What Stu is saying is that today we "do" asanas thoughtfully, whereas the earliest asanas "did us," without any thought whatsoever. In every asana we perform we're consciously or unconsciously looking to find our way back to a time when we were in immediate contact with our deepest divine power.[15]

» *What does the word* asana *mean?*

The Sanskrit word *asana* is nowadays usually rendered as "pose" or "posture," but this isn't its literal meaning. As with many Sanskrit words in the yoga lexicon, the full meaning of this word is impossible to capture in a single English word. In one sense it means "seat," a definition that takes us back to the original application of the word, maybe 2,500 years ago.

Once upon a time, an asana was literally a "steady seat" (*sthiram asanam*), or raised platform, where a yogi sat for meditation. Tradition dictated that this platform be erected in a "clean place" (*shuchau desha*), neither "too high nor yet too low," and covered with a special kind of grass, a cloth, and the hide of a deer or tiger (*Bhagavad Gita* 6.11). There were practical considerations for these requirements. A clean place of course minimized environmental distractions. Since the yogi meditated out of doors exposed to the elements, he needed a platform high enough to raise him off the ground, which might be wet or cold or creeping with creepy things, but not so high that a misstep would send him tumbling disastrously head over heels. The grass, cloth, and skin padded his bottom during what were probably long meditation sessions. In those distant days there weren't more than a handful of poses in the yogi's repertoire, and all of them were seated poses, the most enduring of which was Lotus (*padma*).

What is usually lost in translation, however, are two further definitions of asana, "halting, stopping" and "abiding, dwelling." These remind us of the difference between asana and simply "sitting." Everyday sitting is replete with fidgeting and slumping and getting up to go to the bathroom. But when sitting in asana we "stop" all movement and "abide" in our place. This latter word means "to wait patiently for" and "continue to be sure or firm," which echoes Patanjali's famous criteria for a well-realized asana, that the position should be "steady and comfortable" (YS 2.46).

Asana isn't the only name the old books use for a pose. Others include sthana ("standing"), pitha ("seat"), vishtara ("sitting on a seat; reclining on a bed"), and nishadana ("sitting").

» Are asanas always physical?

No, not always. Asana can also be a "mental pose." Though it literally means "seat" or "sitting," nowadays the word *asana* is typically translated as "pose" or "posture." This of course reflects the popular notion that an asana is some kind of formalized arrangement of the physical body in space, of which there are hundreds of examples and variations. But every now and then we find in one of the old texts a rather different interpretation of the practice.

In the twelfth-century *Tracks of the Adepts' Doctrine* (SSP 2.34), asana isn't ultimately physical at all, though the text advises a yogi to initially assume an appropriate sitting pose to establish a foundation for practice. The real "seat" (*asanna,* note the alternate spelling) is to, in effect, "sit" in "one's true or original state or nature," *svarupa,* the exact word Patanjali uses to name the Self (YS 1.3). A commentary on this passage explains that:

> [An] asana is much more than a mere body posture. Its emphasis is on a mental posture or mental attitude . . . a fixation of the mind in its characteristic form, i.e. *cinmatra* ("sheer consciousness"). . . . [The] body posture is only a help in achieving the mental pose. . . ."[16]

We can find more examples of this reinterpretation of the meaning of asana in a few of the Yoga Upanishads. The dating of this loose collection of twenty-one books is problematic, but generally speaking we can situate them sometime from the fourteenth to the fifteenth century. As does the *Siddha Siddhanta Paddhati,* they remind us that the Self or Brahman, the Absolute, is the true "seat." There's a beautiful passage in the *Radiant Point Upanishad* (*Tejo Bindu Upanishad* 3.22–25) that describes this (and which we might use as a meditation in preparing for a physical asana practice):

I shine by myself; I am my own Atman, my own goal, enjoy myself, play in myself, have my own spiritual effulgence, am my own greatness and . . . am in myself happily seated (*sukha asina*). . . . Sitting on the real throne (*simha asana*) of my own Atman, I think of nothing else but my own Atman.

The *Triple Tuft Brahmana Upanishad* (*Tri Shikhi Brahmana Upanishad* 28–32) reinterprets all the limbs of the Classical Yoga practice in a similarly symbolic manner:

Detachment in relation to the body and the organs of sense, is known . . . as *Yama*. Attachment towards the ultimate Truth continuously is known as *Niyama*. The state of indifference to all things is the best Posture [*Asana*]. The faith in the falsehood of all this world is the control of the vital airs [*Pranayama*]. . . . The facing inward of the citta (mind) is *Pratyahara*. The stagnant state of the citta, they know as the holding of *Dharana*. The reflection that "I am absolute consciousness alone," is known as *Dhyana*. The perfect obliteration of the sense of Dhyana is known as *Samadhi*.

An old tantric text named after the mythic "cow of plenty," the *Kamadhenu Tantra* (31), does something to the word *asana* that we've also seen done to the words *hatha* and *guru*. That is, it separates *asana* into its three constituents, *a-sa-na*, and assigns each a meaning that, when taken together, neatly summarizes the three goals of Hatha Yoga: *a* is *atma samadhi,* the "putting together with the self" or Self-realization; *sa* is *sarva roga pratibandha,* the "prevention of all disease"; and *na* is *siddhi prapti,* the "obtaining of supernormal powers."

Finally, there's a symbolic "seat" often located between the eyebrows. Various names are given to this spot, the so-called third eye, among them: the wisdom eye (*jnana cakshus* or *netra*), Shiva's stand (*shiva sthana*), and the wheel of command (*ajna cakra*).

» *Why do we practice asanas?*

Modern students no doubt have their own ideas about why we practice asanas. Most of us do so for reasons of health, whether mental or physical.

We may want to relieve the common stresses and strains of daily life or to stay in physical shape, or we may use asana as a kind of therapy for various injuries and conditions.

The old yogis, too, had very specific reasons for their practice. They strongly believed that asanas have a salutary effect on the physical body, and that practice frees us from the physical distractions and limitations of poor health, thereby establishing a hospitable environment for further training. Similarly, asana was thought to "destroy death," to extend the practitioner's life, to give him/her the precious time needed to complete the arduous training and gain liberation. They also believed that asana stokes the "fire in the belly," which improves digestion and elimination, and strengthens (or as they said, "bakes") the body in preparation for pranayama and meditation.

There's even more. As we have seen, the old yogis believed that our physical body is supported by a subtle body that's invisible to the human eye but readily apparent to the "eye of wisdom" (*jnana cakshus*), better known as the "third eye." This subtle body is crisscrossed by a network of thousands of energy channels (*nadi*) that transport vital energy (*prana*) to every nook and cranny. In the average person these channels gradually "silt up," due to poor posture, ill health, and stress, preventing prana from flowing freely. Asanas, the yogis say, will dredge out these blocked channels so that prana can be used in the service of yoga, especially to assist with awakening of kundalini (see below) and the realization of our authentic being.

» How many asanas are there in Hatha Yoga?

> There are as many asanas as there are species of living beings. [Only] the great lord [Maheshvara, i.e., Shiva] knows all their varieties. Of the 84 lakhs, one for each has been mentioned. So Shiva has created 84 seats (*pitha*) [for yogis].
>
> *Goraksha's Tracks* (*Goraksha Paddhati*) 1.8–9

The traditional number of asanas in Hatha Yoga can be traced back at least to the twelfth century C.E. and a book titled *Goraksha's Tracks*. In it we're told that Shiva, the divine source and "patron saint" of Hatha Yoga, counted out eighty-four lakhs of asanas, as many as there are "species of living beings" in nature. Now a lakh is an Indian measure that equals one hundred thousand, which when multiplied by eighty-four results in the staggering total of 8,400,000 asanas. It goes without saying—but I'll say it anyway—that this number shouldn't be taken literally. Like the forty days and nights of rain in the Genesis flood story, 8.4 million simply represents a very large, indeterminate number.

> Of these, 84 are most "excellent," of which 32 are auspicious (*shubha*) in the world of humans.
>
> *Gheranda Samhita* 2.2

Shiva might know all the varieties of asanas, as *Goraksha's Tracks* states, but he's a god after all; dealing with over eight million poses is certainly not humanly possible. So as a favor to us, Shiva culled from all the poses a much more manageable eighty-four asanas. This he did by selecting the most "excellent" (*vashishtha*) representative asana from each lakh (though why these were so judged is nowhere explained). Besides *Goraksha's Tracks,* I found five more old Hatha texts that mention the number eighty-four: *Gheranda Samhita* (2.1), *Hatha Ratna Avali* (3.7, 8, 23), *Shiva Samhita* (3.96), *Joga Pradipyaka* (chapter 3), and *Hatha Yoga Pradipika* (2.2) (the ten-chapter version, published by the Lonavla Yoga Institute). Oddly, or so it seems to me, four of these books don't feel compelled to name all eighty-four poses; in fact, the *Goraksha Shataka* and the *Shiva Samhita* only include two and four asanas respectively, all of the sitting variety. The oldest of the six books, the *Hatha Yoga Pradipika,* describes fifteen asanas, and the *Gheranda Samhita* singles out the most "auspicious" thirty-two poses.

We might pause here briefly to wonder, by what standard are Gheranda's thirty-two asanas judged to be auspicious? The text itself offers no obvious suggestions, and thirty-two isn't your typical meaning-laden symbolic number, like, say, nine or twelve, nor does it seem to be significantly related in any way to eighty-four. I did turn up one curious numerical parallel, however. In the first chapter of the *Hatha Yoga Pradipika* (1.5–9), we find Svatmarama's roster of thirty-two "great adepts" (*maha siddhas*). This is a lineage of yogis, beginning with Shiva, who've "broken

Time's staff" (*kala danda,* an emblem of the god of death, Yama) and freely wander about in "Brahma's egg" (*brahma anda*), which is yoga talk for "the universe." In other words, they've conquered both time (and so death) and space. Does the thirty-two in Svatmarama's work have an echo in the thirty-two of Gheranda's? We might guess that it does, but it's only speculation.

So only two of the six traditional books of Hatha Yoga name all eighty-four asanas, and neither of these actually describes all of the poses named. Thus from the oldest texts of the tradition we have descriptions for only thirty-six asanas (from the HRA), leaving us in the dark about the remaining forty-eight. How, for example, does one perform the Decorative Pose (*shilpasana*)? The Ether Pose (*akashasana*)? How about the Gem Pose (*ratnasana*)? Even the *Encyclopedia of Traditional Asanas,* compiled by the Lonavla Yoga Institute in Lonavla, India, which includes nearly a thousand asanas, hasn't a clue. There's only one traditional Hatha Yoga book that both names and describes all eighty-four asanas, the comparatively recent *Joga Pradipyaka.* What, exactly, is going on here?

It turns out that just as the number 8,400,000 isn't to be taken literally, the number eighty-four is also something of a smokescreen. It's widely accepted in the yoga world that this number has symbolic significance. S. Dasgupta, in *Obscure Religious Cults* (1946), cites numerous instances of variations on eighty-four in Indian literature that stress its "purely mystic nature";[17] the mendicant Ajivakas, for example, believes the soul must pass through 840,000 stages before it lands in a human body. Gudren Bühnemann, in her comprehensive *Eighty-four Asanas in Yoga,* notes that the number "signifies completeness, and in some cases, sacredness."[18]

Some writers try to explain the import of eighty-four by pointing out that it's a product of other recognizably symbolic or sacred numbers, such as seven and twelve. For John Campbell Oman, in *The Mystics, Ascetics, and Saints of India* (1905), seven represents the number of so-called classical planets in Indian astrology (the Sun and Moon, Mercury, Venus, Mars, Jupiter, and Saturn), and twelve, the number of signs in the zodiac. What the asanas have to do with astrology though, isn't explained. Matthew Kapstein gives seven and twelve a slightly different spin, noting that from a "numerological point of view," both are related to three and four, the former as the sum of the two numbers (3 + 4 = 7), the latter as the product (3 x 4 = 12). By then multiplying the sum by the product, we arrive at our eighty-four. Kapstein remarks that symbolically eighty-four "encompasses the range of possible relationships obtaining among the innumerable magical and natural categories involving threes and fours," though unfortunately he doesn't provide any specific examples. However, from a "historical perspective," he concludes, eighty-four is "entirely arbitrary."[19] Nevertheless, taking our cue from Bühnemann, we can be fairly confident in assuming that the number is a "code," signaling to yoga insiders that the asanas, however many there actually are, are more than mere physical exercises, that each is part of a "complete" or holistic system of "sacred" practices.

> Eighty-four asanas were spoken of by Shiva. Of these I'll describe the four that "consist of the best" (*sara bhutan*).
>
> *Hatha Yoga Pradipika* 1.33

Are we done paring down the asanas yet? No, not quite. Where the *Gheranda Samhita* extracted the thirty-two most auspicious asanas from eighty-four, Svatmarama (who includes only fifteen asanas in the *Hatha Yoga Pradipika* while noting the number eighty-four only in passing) makes the more radical cut to the four "best." Why four? Based on its association with the square and the directions of space, four (like eighty-four) is a very significant number in yoga. The square stands for the "earth" element, the densest of the five traditional elements (along with earth, water, fire, air, and ether) that compose matter, both subtle and gross. Four then signifies solidity and stability on the one hand, and wholeness or totality on the other (that's why several of the old yoga books, like the *Yoga Sutra* and *Vedanta Sutra*, have four chapters, to express their "completeness" as a system). I suppose the message here is that these four asanas in some way are the foundation of all the asanas. Of course, with all of these numbers there's a chance that I'm reading into them a meaning that was never intended by the authors of these books—that they had something else entirely in mind by choosing these numbers, or that they had nothing in mind at all, and the numbers were simply picked out of a hat.

In any case, do you want to try to guess which asanas are included among the four "best"? When I ask this question of unsuspecting students they usually answer with the poses they're most familiar with and practice frequently. Head Stand and Shoulder Stand, for example, the "king" and "mother" of the asanas in Iyengar method, are popular responses, as are assorted backbends and standing poses. But this is traditional, not modern Hatha Yoga we're talking about. The focus, remember, isn't on asana, but pranayama and meditation.

So it's only to be expected that all four of the "best" asanas are sitting poses, which usually comes as quite a shock to most students. But once given this hint, there are two that are pretty easily guessed, Lotus (*padma*) and Adept (*siddha*). The third asana isn't immediately obvious, but by a process of elimination one of my students usually comes up with Auspicious (*bhadra*), a pose we nowadays know as Bound Angle (*baddha kona*). It's the fourth "best" pose that gives everyone fits, which leads me to suspect it's not among the Top Forty on asana practice charts. What is it? The Lion (*simhasana*), honored (*pujita*) by eminent yogis, presumably because, according to Svatmarama, it unites the three main bonds (*bandha*) and so is centrally important in pranayama (HYP 1.52).

Done? Nope, still one more to go: the supposed best of all poses. Here we see a process that's not uncommon in the yoga tradition: you start with a mind-blowingly large number and gradually pare it down until only one is left standing. Hint: it's one of Svatmarama's four "best" poses. Given its iconic role in the yoga world, we might reasonably imagine that Lotus is the most prized, but no, that distinction goes to Adept, at least according to Svatmarama. Among the asanas, he claims it's *mukhya*, "first, principal, chief," as it purifies the body's subtle energy channels (*nadi*) and ultimately breaks open the door to liberation (*moksha*). (He also assures us that Lotus counters all disease, and favors the practitioner with *bodham atulam*, "unequalled knowledge," and ultimately, liberation—not bad for a second-best "best" asana.)

» Is it true that the Shoulder Stand used to be a mudra?

The word "repurpose," according to my dictionary, first showed up in our language around 1984. It means to take something that was designed for one purpose and, perhaps when it becomes worn out or obsolete, apply it to a new purpose. For example, I have a couple of ball-shaped, one-pound, lead fishing weights. I'm not entirely sure what fishermen and women use these for, but I'm pretty sure it's not the same thing as I do. When I'm in Corpse (*shava*) I lay the weights in my upturned palms to help soften the roots of my thumbs.

Now the word has only been around for thirty years, but humans have been repurposing things for a very long time, and yogis are no exception. So yes, it's true that Shoulder Stand (*sarvanga*) started out as a *mudra* (see "What's a mudra?" on page 200). This pose and two other well-known asanas, *utkata* and *pashcimottanasana*, have all been repurposed.

INVERTED ACTION SEAL
(*VIPARITA KARANI MUDRA*, HYP 3.77–82; GS 3.29–32)

> Navel up, palate down, Sun up, Moon down. This is named "inverted action" (*viparita karani*) [seal].
>
> *Hatha Yoga Pradipika* 3.79

Five-and-a-half centuries ago, the asana we call Shoulder Stand today was instead counted among the mudras and known as *viparita karani mudra,* "inverted action seal" (we'll be getting to the mudras shortly). Like its soul mate, Head Stand, Shoulder Stand is no doubt one of modern yoga's most iconic poses. Mr. Iyengar calls it the "Mother of asanas." At the end of his detailed instructions for the pose in *Light on Yoga*, he spends an entire page listing its many supposed benefits, devoting more space to the pose than any other in the book save Head Stand. According to Mr. Iyengar, Shoulder Stand aids proper functioning of the thyroid and parathyroid glands, relieves ailments like asthma and bronchitis, hypertension, insomnia, and ulcers, cures headaches and common colds . . . and the list goes on. All these may be reason enough to practice this pose regularly (though many of the benefits are anecdotal and haven't been medically verified), but back in the day the yogis had one and only one goal in performing this exercise, and it's nowhere to be found in Iyengar's list. What was it?

We run across many strange ideas in the old yoga books, ideas that are hard for us modern Westerners to understand. This one involves a mysterious subtle organ, usually located at the base of the brain or back of the throat, that exudes the priceless elixir of immortality (*amrita,* literally "no death"). Just as each of us is said to carry hidden in our body the potentially limitless transformative energy of kundalini, so also, according to the yogis, each of us is supplied with a reserve of elixir that, if used properly, will extend our lives far beyond the normal span of years. The problem is that we're all, unconsciously at least, wastrels, letting our precious fluid of immortality drip through our proverbial fingers. It seems our normal posture is the culprit; that just by being upright our precious elixir trickles down from its source in the head into the belly, where it's vaporized in the furnace of the solar plexus.

The solution—"cheating the Sun's mouth" (*suryasya vancanam*) as the *Hatha Yoga Pradipika* (1.78) calls it—is remarkably simple. The yogis, ever innovative, merely flipped themselves topsy turvy: "Sun up," that's the belly, "Moon down," that's the head. With the usual relationship of head and belly reversed in inverted action, the amrita is preserved. And the yogis who learn to drink their fill of it, writes Svatmarama, break the punishing rod of time, conquer death, and ramble about the universe, "Brahma's Egg" (*brahma anda*), at will.

Before you start upping your practice of Shoulder Stand to a rigorous five minutes a day, I should mention one little snag. According to the *Hatha Yoga Pradipika*, the pose should be held for one *yama*, an "eighth part of a day"—or as we like to say, three hours. Now is there any record of anyone ever holding Shoulder Stand for this length of time? The answer, believe it or not, is yes and no.

Yes, because a modern yogi did hold a topsy-turvy pose for three hours. But no, because it wasn't Shoulder Stand but rather Head Stand. The practitioner in question was the American yogi and explorer Theos Bernard (1908–1947). He writes about his experience in a book published the year of his death, titled *Hatha Yoga*. It seems that the brevity with which the old yoga texts described *viparita karani*—again "Sun up, Moon down"—allowed Bernard to take a different interpretation of the pose's performance. Nonetheless, he was still upside down for three hours a day.

According to Bernard's account, the first week he held Head Stand for ten seconds every morning, then added thirty seconds each week until, after several months, he reached fifteen minutes. At this point he added an evening practice of the same duration, which gave him thirty minutes daily. After a month he added a noon practice, and increased all three practices to twenty minutes, achieving thereby an hour daily. Eventually he dropped the noon practice and focused on increasing the time of the morning and evening practices until, ultimately, the morning practice topped out at three hours and the evening practice could be dropped.

So, did it work? Did Bernard live to a ripe old age? We'll never know. On a search for rare manuscripts in northern India in 1947, Bernard and his travelling party were reportedly attacked by local tribesmen. His body was never found, and Bernard was never heard from again. He was thirty-nine years old.

YOGA STORY

The Churning of the Ocean

Whatever nectar flows from the moon (whose form is divine) is swallowed by the sun. Consequently the body ages.

Hatha Yoga Pradipika 3.77

Drench the body with nectar from the head to the soles of the feet. One will definitely get a great body, and great strength and heroism.

Hatha Yoga Pradipika 4.53

Once upon a time, the thirty gods and their world were abandoned and cursed by the bad-tempered and slightly nutty sage Durvasas, who was a portion of the god Shiva. The plants withered and the people became greedy and weak. The demons saw their chance and attacked the gods who, in their vulnerability, ran for help to their beloved grandfather, Brahma. He told them, "Go to Vishnu, the All-Pervader, who destroys demons and dispels suffering." So off went the gods to find Vishnu on the shore of the Milk Ocean.

When they reached Vishnu, who had his conch, discus, and mace in hand, the gods prostrated at his feet and praised him profusely. Pleased, Vishnu explained what to do: "Take these herbs and toss them into the Milk Ocean to make the immortal nectar (*amrita*), the essence of life. Using Slow Mountain (*mandara*) as a churning stick and the serpent-king Vasuki as a churning rope, stir the ocean. Tell the demons that if they help they'll be rewarded just like you. But know that I will arrange it so that only you, the gods, and not the demons, obtain the immortal nectar."

So the gods tossed the herbs into the Milk Ocean, whose glow, it was said, "was as clear as the sky in autumn." Then they grabbed the tail of the serpent-king Vasuki, while the demons took hold of his head. The fiery hot hissing of the snake's mouth sapped the demons of energy, while the rain clouds that emanated from his tail refreshed the gods. Thus began the epic event known as the "ocean stirring" (*samudra mathana*).

In the middle of the Milk Ocean, Vishnu assumed the form of one of his avatars, Kurma the Tortoise, and supported on his back the great churning-stick mountain. Now many marvelous things began to rise out of the ocean, treasures known as the "Fourteen Jewels" (*chaturdasha ratnam*). There was Surabhi (or Kamadhenu), the sacred cow, who could feed countless people with her milk; Airavata, the elephant with four tusks, and the white horse Uchchhaih Shravas; Varuni (or Mada), goddess of wine; sweet-smelling Parijata, the tree of paradise, and Kalpa Vriksha, the wish-fulfilling tree; the Apsarases, the celestial nymphs, "matchless in grace, perfect in loveliness"; Shankha, the victory conch, Gada, the mace of sovereignty, and Dhanus, a magic bow; Chandra, the "cool-rayed" Moon; Kalakuta (or Halahala), a virulent poison; Shri (also called Lakshmi), the goddess of love, beauty, and prosperity (who was to become Vishnu's wife); and finally there appeared Vishnu's physician, Dhanvantari, carrying the most precious gift of all, the jar (*kumbha*) of the immortal nectar.

The demons stole the jar from Dhanvantari, but Vishnu immediately tricked them with an illusion: he turned himself into a beautiful woman named Mohini, who distracted the demons, stole back the jar, and gave it to the gods. The gods drank of it, and with their newfound power they defeated the demons, who scattered to the winds and to the netherworld. The gods rejoiced and praised Vishnu, and the world and all its people were gloriously restored.

Immortal doesn't belong only to the gods. Each of us has a supply that can be accessed through certain yoga practices. Different texts say it's stored in different places, usually the Palate Wheel (*talu chakra*), associated with the uvula, at the back of the throat, or the Thousand-Spoked (*sahasrara*) center at the crown. In any case, in the average person, Immortal drips into the Jeweled City Wheel (*manipura chakra*), located at the navel, where it's incinerated in the fires of the solar plexus. Because we waste our supply of Immortal, we slowly age and eventually die. The *Shiva Samhita* (2.6–11) suggests there are two kinds of Immortal:

> In this body . . . there is the nectar-rayed moon . . . on the top of the spinal cord. . . . This has its face downwards, and rains nectar day and night. The ambrosia further sub-divides itself into two subtle parts: One of these, through the channel named Ida, goes over the body to nourish it, like the waters of the heavenly Ganges. . . . This milk-ray (moon) is on the left side. The other ray, brilliant as the purest milk and fountain of great joy, enters through the middle path (called Sushumna) into the spinal cord, in order to create this moon. At the bottom of Meru [the spine] there is the sun. . . . In the right side path (Pingala) the lord of creatures carries (the fluid) through its rays upwards. It [i.e., the sun] certainly swallows the vital secretions.

Immortal is also called "juice" or "extract" (*soma*), "ease" or "comfort" (*sudha*), "immortal liquor" (*amara varuni*), "milk" or "nectar" (*piyusha*, the drink of immortality produced at the churning of the ocean of milk), and "not aging" (*nirjara*).

EXCESSIVE (*UTKATA*, GS 2.27)

> Fix the balls of the feet on the ground and lift the heels off the ground, then squat down on the raised heels. This is called *utkatasana*.

> Paraphrase of *Gheranda Samhita* 2.27

The Sanskrit word *utkata* means "exceeding the usual measure, immense; richly endowed with; drunk, mad, furious; excessive, much; superior, high, proud; uneven; difficult." These are a lot of words to choose from to render *utkata* into English. I translate it as "excessive" on account of *utkata's* root, *kata,* which means "excess" (among other things). As you may know, the Excessive Pose (*utkatasana*) is a kind of semi-squat, which B. K. S. Iyengar compares to "sitting on an imaginary chair," though to be more precise, it's more like sitting on the edge of a tall stool. It's supposed to benefit the shoulders, chest and back, legs and ankles, and the heart and abdominal organs; "Horsemen" are said to benefit from the pose, and I assume this not a mystical analogy but a reference to men (and presumably women) who ride horses.

What most students probably *don't* know is that this staple pose of modern yoga is a rather more friendly version of a traditional yoga asana that can be traced all the way back to at least the mid-fifteenth-century *Hatha Yoga Pradipika* (though it's only mentioned, and not described, at 2.26). According to *Gheranda Samhita* (2.27), the traditional Excessive is a full-blown squat with the heels lifted off the ground to support the buttocks, so the practitioner balances on the balls of the feet, no doubt somewhat precariously at first.

You might imagine, given the differences between the modern and traditional expressions of this posture, that the original purpose of the pose differed from the purpose outlined by Iyengar, and you'd be right. In fact, forget about riding horses and all the rest of it. The origin of Excessive Pose is revealed in the first chapter of the *Gheranda Samhita* (1.44–46), in the section on the "six cleansing methods" (*shat karma shodana*), specifically the subsection on "water bladder" (*jala basti,* also spelled *vasti,* see HYP 2.26–28). Here we learn that the pose is assumed in preparation for an enema, one small step in the elaborate physical cleansing process dictated for new practitioners. We're instructed to squat as described above in water up to the navel, and insert a "hollow tube" (*nala,* typically made of bamboo or reed, and three inches long) in you-know-where, then continually contract and dilate the sphincter. This, asserts the anonymous author of the *Gheranda Samhita,* is supposed to prevent urinary disease (*prameha*), constipation (*guda varta*), and gas (*krura vayu,* literally "ferocious wind"). But there's something even better. As a result of this purge, we become like *kama deva,* the Hindu god of love, with a body of "our own choice." Svatmarama, too, extols the blessings of water bladder to prevent an enlarged spleen and purify the senses, but disappointingly says nothing about a god of love.

Intense Stretch of the West
(*PASHCIMOTTANASANA* or *PASHCIMA UTTANASANA*, GS 2.26)

From very early on in my yoga career, I was taught that the sitting forward bend known as *pashcimottanasana* meant the "intense stretch" (*uttana*) of the "west side" (*pashcima*) of the body. In Hatha Yoga's mythic geography of the body, the "west" is the entire back of the body, while the "east" (*purva*) is the front (and so gives us *purva uttanasana*). There was no reason to question this interpretation as the "intense stretch" I felt when in the pose, at least along the backs of my legs, was certainly proof enough of its validity.

But when I began to study the traditional texts, I came upon a description of this pose that gave an entirely different interpretation to the word *pashcima*. The word didn't name the back of the *body* at all; instead, it referred to what's called the "western path" (*pashcima marga*), which is a synonym for the "most gracious channel," the *sushumna nadi*. This most important channel is said to pass through the spinal canal. Though it's rather challenging for many modern practitioners, in the old days the yogi could fairly easily lay his front torso down on his legs. The pressure on the belly resulting from its contact with the thighs is said to force the prana to the base of the spine and into the sushumna (pashcima marga).

So the original intent of pashcimottana wasn't so much to stretch the back of the body, but to serve as a sitting position for pranayama. In fact, there's a verse in the eighteenth-century *Moonlight on the Principles of Hatha* (*Hatha Tatva Kaumudi*, 7.41) that names this pose *pashcimatana bandha,* the "western bond." This directly allies the pose with that subset of mudras known as *bandhas,* three of which are central to the practice of pranayama (we'll come to these exercises shortly).

The somewhat later *Joga Pradipyaka* (3.69–77) goes even further. It instructs us to sit "facing north" in the pose and "practice pranayama to fill the sushumna with air."

Secret Lives of Asana

As we see with *guru* and *hatha,* Sanskrit words often have more than one interpretation, whether that's literal or figurative. Many of the asana names, both traditional and modern, have "secret lives," something "hidden" in them that isn't well known, which adds another layer of meaning to their names and so deepens our appreciation for the poses. Here are four to consider.

STAFF (*DANDA*)

Staff (*danda*) is the basic sitting pose; it's to the seated poses what Mountain (*tada*) is to the standing poses. We usually translate *danda* as "staff," an image that compares the central support of our body, the spine, to the staff of the wandering yogi, which supplies him with support and stability. In this sense then, the staff-spine reminds us of traditional yoga's strict asceticism. (The spine is also called the "staff of Meru," *meru danda*, which then analogizes it with Mount Meru, the great mountain at the hub of the Hindu mythic universe.)

What's usually overlooked, though, is that *danda* also means "scepter," a symbol of royal power and sovereignty, which represents the other side of the yoga coin. Along with the sacrifice of worldly goods and relationships, the yogi acquires king-like eminence and power; for example, in the dialogue that opens *Gheranda Samhita*, the disciple Canda calls the guru Gheranda "king of yoga," *yogesja*, and "lord of yoga," *yogeshva*.

So remember, in each and every yoga pose there are two roles to play. First, you're the penniless, solitary ascetic slowly making your rounds from town to town, begging for your food, everything you own is packed on your back, in tireless pursuit of the Real and the True. Second, in sharp contrast to the solitary, you are the glorious ruler of a great nation, seated on a throne wielding a scepter of unlimited power.

BRIDGE (*SETU*)

We usually translate *setu* as "bridge," a word that's quite descriptive of the shape of the pose it names (there are two *setu* poses in the Iyengar system, see LoY, *setu bandha sarvangasana*, 258, and *setu bandhasana*, 296). A bridge, of course, joins two places separated by a gap or an obstacle. But *setu*, paradoxically, also means "dam" or "dike," which is a barrier of some kind, usually built across a watercourse to hold back water.

Now in certain of the Vedic Upanishads (especially CU 8.4.1–2, translation following by R. Radhakrishnan), setu is used as an image of the Self, which then is said to serve as both a dam and a bridge between the mundane and divine worlds. As a dam the Self keeps the two worlds apart, so that between them "cross neither day, nor night, nor old age, nor death, nor sorrow. . . . All evils turn back therefrom." This, it seems, keeps the divine from being polluted by the slings and arrows of the mundane, though we might expect the divine to be a little bit more open and compassionate to the folks on the other side of the wall.

Conversely, the Self is also a bridge, but only those "who practice the disciplined life of a student of sacred knowledge" can cross it. In crossing, if a person is "wounded, he becomes no longer wounded, if afflicted, he becomes no longer afflicted."

EAGLE (*GARUDA*)

Garuda is usually rendered as "Eagle," which is good enough, but not quite accurate. Garuda is an eagle—actually an eagle god, the mount of Vishnu—but the word literally means "devourer" because when he was born (after five hundred years in his egg) he was so blindingly radiant that, as my dictionary notes, he was "originally identified with the all-consuming fire of the sun's rays." Alain Danielou has a different take on the name, which he derives from *gr,* "to speak." Danielou writes that Garuda represents the mystical utterances of the Veda, the "magic words on whose wings man can be transported from one world to another with the rapidity of light."[20]

CORPSE (*SHAVA*)

To understand the "secret" of *shava,* we first need a very brief Sanskrit review (you can skip ahead if you've read Chapter 2; if not this will serve as a lesson). All standalone *nagari* consonants, remember, are syllables, each one accompanied by an unwritten *a* (pronounced "uh"). So, for example, the *nagari k,* though it's written with a single character, is transliterated to the Roman alphabet as *ka* (pronounced "kuh").

So then we start with the word *Shiva,* the "patron saint" of Hatha Yoga. The yogis say that if you separate Shiva from his will (*iccha*), that is, his Shakti or power, represented by the *i* in his name, an *a* will pop up to replace the missing *i,* and so we'll have the word *shava,* "corpse." This is why the yogis mysteriously say, "Shiva is shava." It's important to realize then that when you're practicing Corpse you're not actually mimicking a dead body; rather, you're taking the role of the great passive witness, unmoving yet completely engaged in the present moment, enthralled by the "play" of consciousness, which is none other than Shakti.

MORE ON CORPSE

Corpse has a second story surrounding it, but if you're a bit queasy about death and dead bodies, you might just want to skip ahead. Apparently, some of the Tantric schools took (and may still take today) the practice of shava quite literally and enlisted the aid of an actual corpse. Interested in trying it out? Well then, once you find a corpse, all you'll need to do is sit astride it, being sure to face north, and draw a geometric design (*yantra*) on its back as you recite different mantras.

Why an actual corpse? As John Woodroffe explains, a corpse is a "pure form of organized matter" that is also, it goes without saying, "free from sin or desire." So the divinity (*devata*) that's been invoked by the Tantric ritual can materialize unhindered "by means of the corpse." If all goes well with the rite, the resurrected corpse will turn its head around and ask the practitioner what he'd like for a boon, which may be "spiritual or worldly advancement as he wishes." Woodroffe adds, unnecessarily it seems to me, that this altogether literal performance of shava is "attended by many terrors." The point of the practice, however, is to overcome fear, master indifference, and, in the "interior cremation ground," burn up the "desire body" (*kamika*) in the "fire of knowledge."[21]

>> *I thought Sun Salutation was said to be thousands of years old, but you have written that it is barely a hundred years old. Which is it?*

The practice of the Surya Namaskara . . . has come down to us from the long distant past.

K. PATABHI JOIS, *Yoga Mala* (1999), p. 34

Surya namaskara is a practice whose origins date far back to the earliest epochs of history.

Swami Satyananda Sarasvati,
Surya Namaskara (1973), p. 4

"Sun Salutation" is a straightforward translation of *surya namaskara.* *Surya,* which derives from *svar,* "to shine" (from which also comes *svarga,* the "world of light" or "heaven"), is one of at least a dozen Sanskrit words for "sun." *Namaskara* consists of two words, *namas,* which means "bow, obeisance, reverential salutation, adoration," and *kara* (from the verb *kr*), which means "to do" or "to make."

I imagine a fair number of yoga students, particularly those who count themselves among the enthusiasts of the *vinyasa* or "flow" style of practice, have at least a passing familiarity with this popular sequence of linked poses (hereafter referred to as Sun). Sun is performed in slightly different ways by different yoga schools. The one I'm most familiar with has thirteen basic "stations," each one consisting of a single pose and, since the last five stations in the sequence mirror the first five in reverse order, with a total of eight poses. In their order of performance, these are: Mountain (*tada*), Raised Hands (*urdhva hasta*), in which the arms are stretched up vertically from the previous pose, Standing Forward Bend (*uttana*), Lunge (one leg stepped back, leaving the other leg bent at a right angle), Downward-Facing Dog (*adho mukha shvana*), Plank, Four-Limb Staff (*caturanga danda*), Upward-Facing Dog (*urdhva mukha shvana*), and then the first five are repeated in reverse order to complete the sequence (which is then repeated reversing the legs in Lunge).

There's no doubt that Indians have, since ancient Vedic times up to the present, venerated the Sun as the "soul of all that moves not or moves" in our world (RV 1.115.1). To acknowledge their dependence on and devotion to its life-giving light and heat, they practice daily rituals which include, among other elements, the recitation of laudatory mantras (drawn from the *Rig, Sama,* or *Yajur Vedas*), offerings of water, rice, and flowers, prescribed hand gestures (*hasta mudra*) and physical movements or postures, such as bowing or standing on tiptoes with arms upraised.

What is in doubt, however, and the source of some controversy, is the origin, age, and performance history of the present-day Sun Salutation.

Some traditionalists maintain that instructions for the sequence can be found in the Vedas. In an interview with Mark Singleton, author of the groundbreaking and highly controversial study of modern yoga, *Yoga Body* (Oxford, 2010), K. Pattabhi Jois, progenitor of the popular Ashtanga Vinyasa style of yoga, claimed a Vedic origin for Sun Salutation, which would make the practice at least three thousand years old. Jois cited a mantra from the *Yajur Veda* as the direct source of his root sequence, lettered A, and a section of the *Rig Veda* as the source for a variation lettered B. But when Singleton tracked down the citations, he found that neither applied in any way to the modern Sun Salutation or its individual movements.[22] He wrote that the "claim that specific gymnastic asana sequences taught by certain . . . schools popular in the West today are enumerated in the *Yajur* and *Rig Vedas* is simply untenable from a historical or philological point of view."[23]

Other traditionalists take a slightly different position regarding the Vedic origins of the modern practice. They readily admit that the actual procedure of what worshipers called "Sun Salutation" in the ninth century B.C.E., to take an example, wasn't the same as what we do in the twenty-first century C.E. They propose, however, that our Sun Salutation practice is nevertheless based on the earliest Sun Salutations in the sense that both practices have a focus on "health and wealth," a focus which has stayed the same since ancient times. Just because no concrete evidence of a Vedic connection to the modern practice has yet been uncovered isn't for them proof positive that such a connection doesn't exist. In their hearts they believe that someday the evidence will be found by someone digging through a stack of forgotten manuscripts in some dusty nook of an off-the-beaten-track Indian library.

While the traditionalists' faith is admirable, it's still difficult to embrace wholeheartedly. None of the traditional Hatha Yoga books that I'm aware of mention Sun Salutation, or even *any* of the poses that typically contribute to the basic sequence. But we might reasonably allow this much: while the ancient rituals were decidedly not the same as our Sun, certain of their movements, such as bowing and standing with the arms raised, are reminiscent of elements of the modern sequence. It's not impossible then that the old-timey practices are distant precursors to our modern Sun. If this is the case, we have then at least an indirect tie to the Vedas.

What riles the traditionalists is the modern scholar's suggestion that, far from being a hoary practice with scriptural roots, it appears that Sun Salutation is actually an invention of the early twentieth century, and so is something less than a hundred years old. The oldest extant text describing what we recognize as Sun Salutation is a little book, *The Ten-Point Way to Health: Surya Namaskara,* published in India in 1928. Its author was Shrimant Balasahib Pandit Pritinidhi (1868–1951), the Rajah of Aundh (at the time of his reign, a princely state in British-controlled India), who was aptly nicknamed *bala sahib,* the "master of power." Singleton credits the Rajah as the "creator of the modern *suryanamaskar* system."[24] For his part, though, the Rajah, who was solidly in the traditionalist camp, insists that the practice "goes back thousands of years,"[25] though he doesn't argue for a Vedic source. All he did, he writes, is modify and "improve" on the "old style,"[26] though he's somewhat vague about what that style was all about.

Joseph Alter, a professor of social sciences at Yale–NUS College in Singapore, says that the Rajah's innovation represents a "hybrid exercise," a combination of asanas and Indian calisthenics, which the Rajah devised and popularized as a means not only for individual self-improvement but also for strengthening, both physically and morally, the Indian society as a whole. Alter comments:

> In the beautiful and harmonized movements . . . [he] clearly saw the harmonized body of a united India polity that would turn, collectively, away from the gross sensations of modern life—sex, drugs, power, pride, prosperity—and toward the pure experience of self-realization.[27]

Not all of the Rajah's contemporaries, by the way, were enthused about this vigorous practice and its patriotic, supposedly morally uplifting goals. One of the most vocal critics was Shri Yogendra (1897–1989), founder of the Yoga Institute in Mumbai. Writing in *Yoga Asanas Simplified* (first published in 1928), he railed against "exercises involving violence, strain or fatigue," specifically the newfangled Sun. Without doubt, Yogendra didn't consider the practice an ancient one, for he criticized it as a "form of gymnastics" cobbled on to the rituals of sun worship by the "ill-informed." Citing a verse in the *Hatha Yoga Pradipika* (1.15), which warns against "laborious work" (*prayasa*) as an obstacle to yoga success, he concludes that Sun Salutation is "definitely prohibited by the authorities."[28] And he wasn't done. In opposition to the Rajah's project (though not naming him directly), Yogendra condemned as "unhealthy" and immoral the "wedlock" of asanas with "other systems of physical training" for the purpose of cultivating strength and patriotism, and he labeled their proponents "pseudo-yogins."[29]

SHRI YOGENDRA AND THE CRYPT OF CIVILIZATION

Be sure to mark May 25, 8113, on your calendar. You'll definitely want to be on hand, if it's still there, for the opening of the Crypt of Civilization, a room-sized "time capsule" in the basement of Phoebe Hearst Hall on the campus of Atlanta's Oglethorpe University (the Crypt occupies a former underground swimming pool). The Crypt was the brainchild of the university president Dr. Thornwell Jacobs (1877–1956), who had visited the Egyptian pyramids sometime in the 1920s and came to the conclusion that ancient civilizations did a bad job preserving their records. As a favor to future historians and archaeologists, he came up with the idea of the Crypt to preserve "memorials of the civilization which existed in the United States and the world at large during the first half of the twentieth century." Thomas Peters (1884–1973), an inventor and photographer, was appointed to supervise the Crypt's construction and serve as its archivist.

First of all, why did Jacobs choose 8113 as the date to reopen the Crypt? When he began work in earnest on the Crypt in 1936, he calculated that 6,177 years had elapsed since the first known date in history, 4241 B.C.E. according to the Egyptian calendar. So taking 1936 as the midpoint, and counting 6,177 years into the future, he arrived at 8113. And next, what did Peters put in this Crypt to memorialize civilization of the mid-twentieth century? Among many other things, he selected audio recordings (including the voices of Franklin Roosevelt, Benito Mussolini, and Popeye the Sailor Man, with his sage "I yam what I yam"), newsreels, a radio, electric light fixtures, games and toys, a typewriter, a cash register, an adding machine, some dental floss and dentures, various kinds of seeds, plastic toys of Donald Duck and the Lone Ranger, and a can of beer, which, after six thousand years of fermentation, would definitely *not* be lite. And, of course, books. Lots of them, in fact—over eight hundred books stored on 640,000 pages of microfilm (and photographed on a camera he invented).

Shri Yogendra's books were chosen by the Crypt's advisory panel to represent mid-twentieth-century yoga. For a while though, it didn't look like it would happen. Yogendra didn't receive Peters's letter requesting copies of his books until late March, 1940, and the Crypt was scheduled to be sealed in late May. This didn't leave much time, especially considering that one book was out of print—and no Bombay press could be found to produce a copy on such short notice—and that shipping books from India during wartime was an expensive and time-consuming proposition. But in the end it all worked out: Yogendra's books arrived at the last minute, were converted to microfilm, and are now sitting in the Crypt at Oglethorpe University, with only a little more than 6,100 years before they see the light of day.

The Crypt was ceremoniously sealed on May 25, 1940. Posted on the stainless steel door is the following message:

> We depend upon the laws of the county of DeKalb, the State of Georgia, and the government of the United States and their heirs, assigns, and successors, and upon the sense of sportsmanship of posterity for the continued preservation of this vault until the year 8113, at which time we direct that it shall be opened by authorities representing the above governmental agencies and the administration of Oglethorpe University. Until that time we beg of all persons that this door and the contents of the crypt within may remain inviolate.

Most of us perform a stripped-down version of the Raja's original routine. He accompanied his movements with both "seed" (*bija*) mantras and mantras based on the different names for "sun" in Sanskrit, both of which recall the ritual recitations intoned by ancient sun worshipers. He devotes two chapters to these mantras, thoughtfully including an "abridged method" of mantra suitable for "members of other faiths,"[30] such as Christians and Muslims.

Sometime in my own distant past one of my teachers (who shall remain nameless) told me that Sun is really meant to pay homage to two suns, the "outer" macrocosmic one at the center of our solar system, and the "inner" microcosmic one, the "light" of our own consciousness.

» Would you discuss the evolution of the use of props?

The use of props in teaching Yoga is unique to the Iyengar School of Yoga. Pupils of the . . . Institute have well accepted their usage. But many may not be aware that teachers from other Yoga Centres differ in their opinion regarding the use of props in teaching and practicing Yoga. Some feel that "props" create habit-forming and dependent pupils, and prevent them from learning to perform the asanas independently.

Introduction to the interview "Use of Props," in *70 Glorious Years of Yogacharya B. K. S. Iyengar* (1990), pp. 391–402

Props teach alignment; but having learnt, we must quickly discard them. This period varies for each person. . . . We will not achieve the optimum effect if we use props continually (in general).

Dr. Krishna Raman, *Yoga and Medical Science* (2003), p. 54

The Merriam-Webster Dictionary defines a "prop" as "something used in creating or enhancing a desired effect." We use props every day for all kinds of reasons, from training wheels on kids' bikes to help them stay upright while they learn to balance, to crutches to help us get around on a broken foot until it heals. But if you're an Iyengar student, or attend classes influenced by his teaching, the word "prop" most likely conjures images of buckled straps, wood or foam blocks, sand bags, folding chairs, stacks of blankets, bolsters, eye bags, and all the other paraphernalia so closely associated with Iyengar Yoga. Of course, if you're not Iyengar inclined, you may be wondering what props are all about.

One thing they're about, of course, is money. According to numbers compiled in a 2005 report by the International Yoga Therapists Association (IYTA), "Yoga Statistics and Demographics," we Americans spent nearly three billion dollars—yes, billion with a *b*—on yoga stuff, more than the gross domestic product of nearly fifty countries (albeit most of these were very small islands). Where did all that money go? Without being specific, the report lists classes, workshops, and conventions, yoga tights and other duds (three-quarters of all yoga students are women), vacations (usually advertised as "retreats"), various media, including videos, books, and magazines, and "equipment" or props. We have to believe that with yoga blankets selling for thirty dollars, bolsters for seventy dollars, and "limited edition" sticky mats for over a hundred dollars, a fairly sizeable chunk of that three billion went to props.

I suspect many Iyengar-ites would say that props are their guru's brainchild, and indeed, most everything we find in Iyengar classes can be credited to or has been inspired by his inventiveness. We even know when and why he first tried a prop. In 1948, as he explains to an interviewer, he was having difficulty with Bound Angle (*baddha konasana*). So he picked up some "heavy stones" he found lying in the street, and practiced the pose with the stones weighing down his thighs. It seems a bit ironic, doesn't it, that the lucrative yoga prop business got its start with a humble, and free, paving stone.

It might then come as a surprise to Iyengar-ites to learn that yoga props go back at least a thousand years. In those days, an asana was still primarily a "seat" or sitting position, like Lotus, assumed for pranayama and/or meditation. Its success was measured by two classical criteria: it had to be "steady" (*sthira*) but not rigid, and "comfortable" (*sukham*) but not floppy (YS 2.46). Since asanas were intended to be held for a considerable length of time—the duration of a yogi's pranayama or meditation practice—a prop that aided the establishment of steadiness and comfort would be of great value. An early-day Iyengar invented such a prop, called a *yoga pattaka,* which is mentioned in the tenth-century C.E. subcommentary on the *Yoga Sutra,* the *Autumnal Clarity on the Categories [of Existence] (Tattva Vaisharadi).*

Now not everyone agrees on the meaning of *pattaka*. Some translators render it as "yoga table" because one definition of a *pattaka* is a "board or plate (especially for writing upon)." Understood this way, the prop is a small "table" with a single short leg, on which the seated yogi rests his arms while practicing pranayama or meditation. Other translators, however, while admitting such an arm-support table exists, maintain that the author of the commentary was referring to a "girdle," another possible translation of *pattaka*. This prop is a long strip of cloth that the Lotus-seated yogi wraps around his legs and lower back as a lumbar support. (When asked where he got the idea for using a buckled strap in a similar way, Iyengar replied that he had seen statues of Lord Narasimha, "Man-Lion," Vishnu's fourth incarnation, with a cloth wrapped around his knees.)

We occasionally see this girdle in drawings of the deity Shiva, the Hatha yogi's head honcho, sitting in meditation. But more often he is depicted with another traditional support prop, of indeterminate but surely considerable age, called a "yoga staff" (*yoga danda*). This is a short, crutch-like instrument that has two possible uses: most commonly, the yogi presses it into one armpit (which is why the prop is also called a *yoga kaksha,* the latter meaning "armpit") as a way to alter nasal dominance before pranayama practice.

It's generally the case that one of our nostrils is dominant at any one time; in other words, one nostril is taking in more air than the other. The yogis have apparently been aware of this for a very long time, but Western medicine didn't catch on until late in the nineteenth century. Dominance switches naturally back and forth between the nostrils throughout the day and night, typically every two to three hours.

So what does this mean for yoga? Tradition tells us to regulate our activities according to which nostril is dominant. Since the right nostril is the solar nostril (*pingala*), we're instructed to do active things when this nostril is open. Conversely, when the left is more open, it's time to quiet down, maybe do some knitting or read some poetry. Directions here can get pretty detailed. For example, when we step out of bed in the morning we're supposed to use the foot on the side of the body belonging to the more active nostril. Any disruption of the normal rhythm of nostril dominance is also thought to be a harbinger of a coming illness.

The second use of the yoga staff is for long meditations. Typically, the yogi would brace it under his chin to keep his head from tipping forward, and falling flat on his face, should he happen to fall asleep during a marathon meditation.

It should be clear from this then that Iyengar didn't invent yoga props per se. His contribution rather was to take the general idea of a prop and run with it, creating an entirely new repertoire with an enormously broadened field of application, especially in the area of yoga therapy. In a 1999 interview for BBC Radio, he acknowledged two sources of inspiration. One was his guru and brother-in-law, T. Krishnamacharya. Back in the 1930s, Krishnamacharya used ropes affixed to a wall when he taught; each "station" had three pairs of ropes: one about head height, one shoulder height, and one just above the floor (these are familiar fixtures at many Iyengar schools). People with diseases the doctors couldn't figure out would come to him, and he would treat them with the help of gentle stretches provided by the ropes. Incidentally, just as Iyengar wasn't the first yogi to use a prop, Krishnamacharya wasn't the first to use ropes. In a nineteenth-century illustrated manuscript *Treasure House of True Knowledge* (*Shri Tattva Nidhi*), there are nine drawings (among a total of 122) of yogis hanging in various odd positions from a rope (including one yogi who appears to be lifting a heavy weight suspended from a rope that he's gripping in his teeth). The positions are even given Sanskrit names, such as the Cockroach (*paroshnyasana*), the Caterpillar (*vrintasana*), and the Asana of Heaven (*svargasana*).

Iyengar's other inspiration was his beloved Patanjali. He was struck by the terminology Patanjali used in the *Yoga Sutra* to describe the two levels of *samadhi*, "with seed, or supported" and "without seed, or unsupported." These terms, he explained, "made me think, 'why not find ways to do asana with support?' . . . I began thinking on his [Patanjali's] ideas and innovated props as 'support' for good performance of asana with ease but without risk."[31]

If the first modern prop was devised in 1948, we might wonder, just out of curiosity, why there aren't any props demonstrated in Iyengar's classic *Light on Yoga*, first published in 1966. It turns out, as he tells it, that it wasn't until 1975 that he began applying props systematically on a large scale. We see a few results of this breakthrough in his next classic, *Light on Pranayama*, published in 1981. Photographs show an incredibly uncomfortable-looking reclining support made out of wooden blocks, a weighted pole hanging from his shoulders, and an elastic bandage eye wrap.

Now not all modern yoga schools use props in their teaching, and the reasons for this vary. It might be simply that the cost of props and/or the room needed for their storage discourages a small school from stocking them. Other schools are "prop-less" because of the style of yoga they teach. For example, the Ashtanga Vinyasa school, and its numerous "flow-like" offshoots, link their poses together and perform them at a relatively rapid pace, so there's little or no time available to prop a pose safely and effectively.

But there are also non-Iyengar teachers who express strong objections to props, contending that rather than enhance a "desired effect," they do just the opposite; they actually impede a student's "progress." They argue that props, particularly when used by beginners, create an over-dependence that a student continues to rely on long after she should be "standing on her own two feet." It's akin to keeping your crutches even after your foot has healed. Better to struggle with the poses early on if need be, the anti-propists avow, because the student is then compelled to face her challenges head-on, unmitigated by the prop-crutch, and so develop understanding and proficiency at a much faster rate.

Naturally, Iyengar scoffs at this objection. Struggle in a pose, he would say, teaches beginners nothing; rather, it leads to pain and discouragement, and, far from "progressing," a student is tempted to drop yoga in frustration. It's ease of performance that matters most and is most attractive to students, and this ease is created and sustained with props. Props add stability to the poses and help instill correct alignment, a big part of the Iyengar system, both of which decrease fear and pain and build confidence and enthusiasm for the practice. They also allow students to stay in a pose longer, which affords an opportunity to investigate and understand it fully.

We won't here take sides in this debate, since both the Iyengar-ites and the anti-propists make good points (though I will admit leaning toward the former camp, especially when it comes to using a stack of blankets as a support in Shoulder Stand). But is there any truth to the accusation that props encourage "habit forming"? Mr. Iyengar replies that responsibility for any such dependence, should it occur, rests with the student, not the props. So how do we know when it's time to let go of a prop? His answer to this is a bit convoluted, but if I read him rightly, it goes something like this: First, the student must physically integrate the "sense of direction, alignment and understanding of the asana" that the prop promotes, which certainly has no fixed timetable. Then, when these three qualities are established in the pose, the student should proceed free of the props, looking back on the feeling of the propped exercise and comparing it with the feeling achieved in the unpropped version. Propped movements of extension, expansion, and circularity must be reinterpreted in the unpropped exercise. Mr. Iyengar concludes: "Compare the right movements with the props to the wrong movements when done independently. Then one realizes the importance of the props and their utility."[32]

In other words (if I'm interpreting this correctly), the student should make an experiment. She should perform the pose in question independently, without a prop, and assess what she experiences in comparison with the "direction, alignment and understanding" achieved in that same pose with the help of the prop. If the former approximates the latter to a high degree, then she's ready to jettison the prop for good *for that pose*; if, however, her experience in the prop-less asana lacks the three "qualities" to a sufficient degree, then she should continue using the prop, periodically repeating the experiment until direction, alignment, and understanding are realized. Iyengar does remark that certain students, such as those who are quite elderly or somehow disabled, may have to use the props permanently.

» *What are the two models of pranayama?*

I've written quite extensively on pranayama in two previous books, *The Yoga of Breath: A Step-by-Step Guide to Pranayama* (2002), and *Pranayama beyond the Fundamentals* (2006), both available from Shambhala Publications. Here then I'll just briefly review the two models of pranayama.

CLASSICAL YOGA PRANAYAMA

The older and simpler model belongs to Classical Yoga. As you might know, this form of yoga is preliminarily defined as the stilling or restriction (*nirodha*) of any and all movements or fluctuations (*vṛtti*) of consciousness (*citta*). These fluctuations can be gross or subtle. The former includes all movements of the physical body, all the fidgetings and scratchings and adjustings we do practically every minute of every waking day. These bodily fluctuations are quieted by learning to sit very still for what we might consider very long periods of time (for many of us that might be not much longer than a few minutes). This stillness, though, can't be forcefully imposed; it must be what Patanjali calls *sukha*, which in this context means "comfortable."

Even when we're sitting comfortably still, though, we're still moving. How? Our breathing movements, the expansion and contraction of our thorax as we inhale and exhale, count, too, as gross fluctuations. So once our sitting position is more or less established, we turn to the breath in Classical pranayama. In it, the attempt is made to quiet the breath as much as possible, even to the point where it spontaneously comes to a stop for some length of time, a rarified state Patanjali calls the "fourth" (*caturtha*, meaning that it follows the three normal phases of inhale, exhale, and the transition between them).

The "fourth" may seem unusual, but it's probably more common than we realize. We've likely all experienced it before, probably unwittingly and unintentionally, in states when we're intently focused on some matter or project before us, or even when we're reading an especially absorbing book.

The slowing or halting of the breath has an added advantage, since it also begins the stilling of the subtle fluctuations of consciousness. This, too, is a familiar phenomenon. How many times have you thought to yourself or been advised in moments of upset or distress to just take a few slow breaths to calm your mind? Classical pranayama works with the same principle. The practice, says Patanjali, eventually frees the yogi's "inner light" (*prakasha*, see YS 2.52), which facilitates meditation.

HATHA YOGA PRANAYAMA

Classical pranayama is a fairly straightforward process that serves as a means to an end, that is, as a way, building on the asana or "steady and comfortable" seat, to further quiet the *vṛttis* in preparation for intense meditation. Hatha pranayama, on the other hand, involves a good deal more than its Classical counterpart. Patanjali covers pranayama in just five sutras out of a total of 195 in the *Yoga Sutra*. Major Hatha books, like the *Hatha Yoga Pradipika* and *Gheranda Samhita*, by contrast, each dedicate a large chunk of an entire chapter to breathing, along with another full chapter on what are indispensable tools for Hatha pranayama, the "seals" (*mudra*) and bonds (*bandha*).

How does Hatha pranayama work? I suppose an entire book or two could be written on this subject—which I've actually done—so here I'll try to be as concise as possible. Prana is, as you might know, an active force that the yogis say pervades the entire universe and supplies the motive power for it and all its living creatures. Its sister force, so to speak, since they both have the same Mother-source, the divine feminine Shakti ("power"), is *kundalini*, the "coiled one." While prana is active and pervasive, kundalini is dormant and wound tightly like a spring ready to unleash its energy. Each one of us is possessed of a spark of this power, which is said to have the capacity, if properly jump-started, to radically transform our lives (we're also cautioned that if improperly aroused, it could well destroy our lives). Traditionally kundalini is pictured as a coiled (*kundala*), sleeping serpent, resting snug in the root cakra at the base of the spine.

I've already gone over the cakras and nadis earlier in this chapter. What's important to know right now is that there's a split in the heart of our being, between the feminine kundalini and her "spouse," the masculine deity Shiva, who longingly waits at the crown center for his beloved's awakening and their reunion.

Now to simplify things as much as possible, the yogi uses his breath, the gross vehicle for the subtle prana (with the support of the three major bandhas, "root" [*mula*], "net bearing" [*jalandhara*], and "flying up" [*uddiyana*]), to stimulate and waken the serpent and drive her up through the central channel (*sushumna nadi*) to the crown, where the two deities (who are in fact aspects of the world ground, Brahman) are reunited.

Like its predecessor, Hatha pranayama has a number of benefits. The *Hatha Ratna Avali* goes into the benefits in great detail. Among many other things, the breathing practices (in no particular order) pacify thirst, relieve fatigue, purify the body, cure certain disorders, stoke the body's digestive fire, pierce the "knots" (see Chapter 5), and last but not least, control lust, but at the same time liberate you from old age and make you look like either a sixteen-year-old or Kama, the Hindu god of love (see HYP 2.47 and 2.54). And as I've already noted, beyond these benefits the practice is essential in the yogi's efforts to stimulate the slumbering kundalini.

Modern yoga is almost entirely focused on the practice of asana, which as far as getting a decent "workout" is concerned isn't really a problem. But across the thousand years leading up to the twentieth century, the focus of Hatha Yoga, as a Self-realization practice, was pranayama. So we read in the fourteenth-century C.E. *Seed of Yoga* (*Yoga Bija*), the yogi who "wants to achieve success in yoga without controlling the prana breaths or without practicing the pranayama . . . is like a person who wants to cross the ocean with the help of a raw earthen pitcher" (verse 77), the consequence of which you don't want to know.

KUMBHAKA ("POT-LIKE")

To head off any confusion, the word *kumbhaka* has a dual meaning in the old texts. A *kumbha* is a "pot," an image commonly used to represent the torso. This analogy is a vestige of the influence of Indian alchemy on Hatha Yoga. Just as the alchemical retort is where the base matter is heated and distilled and transformed into gold, so the yogi's torso is where the prana is collected and heated and used to transform the yogi's invaluable spiritual potential into a reality. So while the word *kumbhaka* can mean pranayama in general, it also has a very specific meaning: the retention of the breath (or *prana*) in the "pot" (or torso).

YOGA OF THE POT (*GHATA*)

Not all Hatha Yoga texts call their practice "Hatha Yoga." The anonymous author of the *Gheranda Samhita* names the torso the *ghata*, which, like *kumbha*, means "pot." He then calls his teaching the "yoga of the pot" (*ghatastha yoga*, 1.2), by which he means not only the body but also the consciousness "contained" in that body.

» *Why do we practice pranayama?*

The old guides list a large number of benefits—physical, psychological, and spiritual—for pranayama. Of course, this list is based on the authors' practical experiences and the collected wisdom of their schools, and can't be considered scientific evidence, at least by our modern Western standards. But some of the reported physical benefits seem tenable and not beyond the reach of most assiduous aspirants. For example, pranayama is said to stoke the gastric fire, which improves digestion and speeds elimination wastes from the body, and appease thirst and hunger so you won't be distracted by these cravings during practice; open the sinuses to allow more air into the body; purify both the gross and subtle energy systems of the body; and cure many diseases and conditions, including nervous disorders, indigestion, cough, and fever.

But we might take some other purported benefits with a grain or two of skeptical salt. For example, Svatmarama notes somewhat enthusiastically that pranayama will make you resemble a teenager again and improve your love life. I've been practicing now for nearly thirty-three years, and I'm afraid I can't lend any credence to this last assertion, though it does strongly encourage me to practice pranayama regularly. Though the jury is still out, I'm also spurred on by claims that pranayama promotes extraordinary mental and physical powers, such as clairvoyance and levitation; engenders indescribable happiness; and awakens the sleeping serpent kundalini, which leads to living liberation (*jivan mukti*), and, best of all, destroys death. "Even Brahma and other gods in heaven devote themselves to practicing pranayama because it ends the fear of death" (HYP 2.39).

Realistically, as a beginning breather, what benefits can you expect from pranayama? It's hard to generalize, of course, because like anything else, what you get out of the practice depends on how much you put into it. To realize any of the benefits it's crucial to commit to a regular practice and cultivate it properly. Also, some students take to the practice like fish to water. If you're in a yogic frame of mind, you could say that these aspirants have good breathing karma. To other students, though, the practice is about as enjoyable as an appointment with the dentist or a letter from the

IRS. So to be on the safe side, it's best to have relatively moderate expectations about your practice, at least for the first year or so—transcendent bliss and eternal life, I would venture, are probably not in the cards. But based on my own experience and the experiences of my students, there are some benefits in particular that you can reasonably anticipate.

It's not unlikely, first of all, that you'll become more aware of, and gain greater control over, your everyday breath. Why is this a benefit? It's well known and widely accepted that your breath and your mental states are closely related, that the former reflects and can be used, to a certain extent, to influence the latter. I suppose we've all, at one time or another, taken a few deep breaths to calm an angry outburst or to suck up a little extra energy when feeling weary. Certainly yoga has recognized the importance of this connection of breath and consciousness (*citta*) for hundreds of years. Svatmarama, for example, writes that "when prana moves, citta [the mental force] moves. When prana is without movement, citta is without movement. By this [steadiness of prana] the yogi attains steadiness" (HYP 2.2). With the instrument of your breath then, you can monitor and modulate your psychic temperature throughout the day, cooling yourself down when the mental mercury rises, and heating yourself up when it drops. Many of my students have reported that pranayama has made them more relaxed overall and increased their store of energy, not only for yoga practice in general, but also for the business of their everyday lives. I have the sense, now that I've developed a fairly consistent awareness of my breath during the day, that I'm practicing pranayama pretty much all the time (at least when I'm awake), and that I can watch myself—and so get to know myself better—from moment to moment, no matter what I'm doing.

If you adopt a regular practice of pranayama, there's also a good chance that your everyday breathing will become slower; in other words, you'll take fewer breaths throughout the day. The benefit here? You'll expend less energy in the lifelong enterprise of breathing, and so have more energy to direct toward other pursuits—such as asana practice. As your breathing slows, it will also smooth out, which is a kind of natural relaxant for the stresses and strains of our breathlessly paced world. All of this is to say that your breathing will become less effortful, more efficient.

» *What's a* bandha?

It isn't widely recognized that Hatha Yoga includes, in addition to asana and pranayama, a third essential category of practices, composed of bonds (*bandha*) and seals (*mudra*). They're said to cure various diseases and "destroy" death, increase the gastric fire, restrain and channel vital energy in the torso and intensify its transformative potency, confer miraculous powers, and awaken kundalini and lead to samadhi and liberation.

It's difficult to succinctly characterize these widely varied practices of bandhas and mudras, but in general they're muscular contractions and/or asana-like positions, pressurings of two body parts—for example, the chin to the chest, the heel to the perineum, the tongue to the palette—and even meditations (*dharana*) on traditional elements, like earth or fire, localized in the body.

The three most important bandhas for pranayama are Root Bond (*mula bandha*), Net-bearer Bond (*jalandhara bandha*), and Upward Bond (*uddiyana bandha*). We'll come back to these after a short detour.

» *What's a* mudra?

Mudra is literally defined as a "seal," in the sense of an instrument used for sealing or stamping something. According to the tenth-century sage Abhinavagupta there are four different types of mudras, which are gestures formed by the whole body, by the hands, by speech (or the mouth or tongue), and in consciousness by thought only.

But like most words in the yoga lexicon, *mudra* has both a literal meaning and esoteric interpretations. In some old guides a mudra is said to be that which gives (*ra*) joy or pleasure (*muda*) to the gods. Others explain a mudra as that which dissolves or melts spiritual bondage (*mu*), or that which seals (*mudranat*) the entire universe in a state of enlightenment.

There are generally three categories of mudra. The most familiar to us includes the hand (*hasta*) mudras. I'm not sure how many of these mudras there are, but *The Mudras of India (Singing Dragon)* (2012), by Cain and Revital Carroll, covers about fifty yoga hand mudras (and a good number more from Indian dance). Traditionally, mudras are symbolic gestures typically used during meditation and pranayama to invoke the deities associated with them, and to manifest certain abstract ideas and qualities. Holding the hands in a certain shape also helps to quiet overactive hands, which might otherwise generate fluctuations (*vrtti*) in consciousness.

The second category of mudras are the body (*kaya*) mudras. As the name suggests these mudras can be formed by various body parts (e.g., the tongue or eyes), assuming various positions (e.g., inverted or reclining), or by performing various actions (e.g., drawing up and hollowing the front abdomen). These mudras are designed to "seal" energy in and channel it through the body, primarily as an aid to awakening the sleeping kundalini, but also according to the *Gheranda Samhita* to ward off old age, disease, and even death, and to lead to *samadhi* and liberation. If you want to read about these exercises in their original texts, see the third chapter in both the *Hatha Yoga Pradipika* and *Gheranda Samhita*, and the fourth chapter of the *Shiva Sutra*.

The third category consists of the consciousness (*citta*) mudras, probably the least familiar to modern students. The best known example is found in the third chapter of the *Gheranda Samhita* in verses 57 through 63, and collectively known as the "five concentrations" (*pancha dharana*). As the name suggests, these are meditations on the five subtle elements of the body, which are (from densest to lightest): earth, water, fire, air, and space (*akasha*). Each is situated at a different area of the body, from the heart to the crown, and each is symbolized by a color (e.g., earth is yellow), a "seed" syllable (e.g., water is *va*), and a deity (e.g., Rudra stands for fire), and each brings with it a special benefit (e.g., the ability to move through space—are you reading this, NASA? Alpha Centauri, here we come).

>> *Sometimes I hear that there are ten forms of* prana, *other times just five. Which number is right? And could you also say a few words about them?*

You obviously know something about *prana*, the subtle force the yogis say permeates the universe and drives it along. The prana "out there" in space is called "primary" (*mukhya*). When we absorb it into our body on an inhalation, it becomes *vyasti*, "singleness," that is, individualized, and spontaneously divides into five specialized energies, each—except for one—localized in a particular body region. The prana in our body is said to be the microcosmic equivalent of the macrocosmic winds.

Prana is composed of two smaller words, *pra,* "forward, forth," and *an,* "to breathe" (which supplies the root for such words as "animal, animate," and both "animosity" and "equanimity"), so literally *prana* means "to breathe forth." All of the translations I've encountered render the word *prana* as "breath," which is acceptable as long as we remember that in a pranayama context, "breath" is a gross vehicle for the subtle prana. The yogis are working with prana through the medium of the breath.

Now technically there are ten types of prana or more precisely, since they're now inside the body, *vayus,* "winds." Most often, however, we only hear about the five main vayus; the other five are considered minor and control funny things like belching, eye blinking, sneezing, yawning, and hiccuping. We'll leave these winds without further comment because, frankly, I really don't know what to say about them.

As far as the main vayus are concerned, each one controls a major body function and (except for one) is localized in a certain area of the body. *Prana vayu* (not to be confused with prana in general) is localized in the chest and is said in some sources to control breathing, in others just inhalation. Its opposite number is *apana vayu,* the "down breath," localized in the pelvis and said to control elimination (in the sources where prana vayu regulates inhalations, apana vayu functions to monitor elimination). The breath that mediates between these two, the "fire in the belly," is the "middle breath," *samana vayu,* which of course controls digestion. The throat is the seat of the "up breath," *udana vayu,* which controls speech. Finally the last, *vyana vayu,* the "circulating breath" (personified as the son of Udana and the father of Apana), is present throughout the body.

Now that we understand something of the forms of prana, we can return to the *bandhas.* They function in pranayama to help contain the inhaled prana in the "pot" of the torso (*kumbha, ghatta*), and to "heat" it in preparation for awakening the slumbering kundalini. Here's how it works.

The torso-pot, where the work of stimulating kundalini takes place, has two openings, one at the throat, the other at the anus. In order to prevent the prana from "leaking" out of the torso pot, these two openings are sealed, the throat by the Net-bearer Bond, the anus by the Root Bond. These two bonds then serve a second purpose. In order to "heat" the retained prana and apana energies, which tend to move apart—prana up, apana down—the throat and root bonds force these vayus to move toward the same place, the navel. They're joined at the navel by samana vayu, which is used to heat them with the pressure-cooker abdominal lift called the Upward Bond. Finally, this heat is directed at the sleeping serpent kundalini, who resides at the base of the spine in the *root cakra* and who is then stimulated to rise through the central energy channel, the *sushumna nadi.*

SANSKRIT WORDS FOR "WIND"

We read in the *Shiva Samhita* (3.3) that "prana has various names," but not all of these are described in the text. Others include (along with *vayu,* "wind"): *vata* ("wind emitted from the body"); *pavana* ("purifier"); *anila* ("wind"); *maruta,* a name related to *marut* ("shining ones"); the storm gods; and *samirana* ("setting in motion," another name for the god of wind).

» *What is* pratyahara?

When we hear the word *pratyahara,* I would imagine most students think immediately of the Classical version, described below. But there are actually three more pratyahara practices, all associated with Hatha Yoga, that have nothing to do with the senses.

CLASSICAL YOGA PRACTICE (YS 2.54–55)

With the body comfortably steadied (or steadied comfortably) in a seated asana and the breath slowed to a crawl or brought to a stop with pranayama, the next step in the Classical Yoga practice is *pratyahara,* literally "to hold back" or "retreat." Pratyahara is the last of the five so-called outer limbs (*antara anga*) of the eight "limbs" (*anga*) of Classical Yoga. At this point the practitioner draws his senses away from the outer world, where they are usually busily occupied, each with its own interest (ears with sound, nose with smell, and so on). This process is often compared to the setting Sun withdrawing its rays into itself, or a tortoise pulling its limbs and head into its shell. Actually a "shell" is a particularly useful image; the practitioner is essentially retreating into himself behind an impenetrable shell or cocoon. If he's ever to quiet the "fluctuations" (*vrtti*) of consciousness, he must first cut himself off from that unceasing *vrtti*-flood, the outside world, which washes over him with all its distractions from every side. By disengaging from the outer world, the yogi is now free to deal with his interior world and the *vrttis* bubbling up from his own unconscious.

It's important to remember about pratyahara that it's NOT the senses that are being withdrawn directly; rather, the practitioner is quieting his mind, and as a consequence the senses follow along. Vyasa compares this situation to a queen bee and her attendants. "Just as bees follow the course of the queen bee and rest when the latter rests, so when the mind stops the senses also stop their activities" (YS 2.54).

We can use our hands or a prop to assist us with the process of quieting the mind, performing what's called the "six-opening seal" (*shanmukhi mudra*)—that is, using our thumbs and fingers to block our ear canals and eyes (see LoY 106). For a modern version of this technique we wrap our head, covering our eyes and ears (but not our nose) with an Ace bandage.

HATHA YOGA PRACTICE

You can find these practices described in the *Shandilya Upanishad*, 1.8.1ff. (one of twenty-one Yoga Upanishads):

1. Instead of quieting his senses, as in the Classical practice, the practitioner is instructed to *transform* all he takes in with his senses—to experience everything, whether good, bad, or indifferent, as Brahman or the Self (see *Shandilya* 1.8.1).
2. The practitioner is instructed to give up the "fruits," that is, the benefits that accrue from performing his prescribed daily observances.
3. The practitioner is instructed to hold the "air," or prana, at the vital "supports" (*adhara*) of the body, and then withdraw it from each of these in turn. The supports are usually sixteen or eighteen

in number. One version of the practice lists them as follows: the big toes, ankles, mid-calves, knees, mid-thighs, groin, navel, mid-chest, throat, soft palate, nose, mid-forehead, and crown, otherwise known as the "aperture of Brahma" (*brahma randra*).

» *The yogis don't "hear" sound the way the average person does. Could you explain how they describe sound?*

Listen. Hear that? Sound is all around us, whether it's just random noise or organized into language or music. Sometimes the babel of modern life seems overwhelming, and if you're like me, you've learned to tune much of it out, if only to protect your sanity. I wonder though: if I learn to selectively ignore much of the unnecessary racket in my life, what effect will this have on my capacity to hear what *is* necessary, not only the sounds coming to me from the outside world, but from my inner world as well? And if I desensitize myself to the sound the world is making, do I do the same with the "sound" I'm making in my everyday thoughts and conversations? Do I thus inadvertently contribute to the very cacophony I'm trying to avoid?

The yogis are avid listeners, and no sound escapes their notice. It's no surprise then that they've elaborated a "science of sound," since they've transformed just about everything available to us through our five senses into a vehicle for self-investigation and self-liberation. Certainly Western science has also studied sound, but only as a material phenomenon; the yogis' preoccupation with sound has taken them beyond the physical realm into the metaphysical. They've discovered that the whole universe is shaped, pervaded, and will ultimately, at the end of its life cycle (*kalpa*), be reabsorbed by sound—or to be more precise, a vibratory power that has both audible and inaudible manifestations.

It may seem contradictory to talk about inaudible sound, though of course we're bombarded all the time with sounds we can't hear because of the inherent limitations of our sense of our hearing. But for the yogis, subsonic and supersonic sounds are still considered audible, since we can hear them if our hearing is amplified with special instruments. Inaudible sound, by contrast, refers to subtle, or what the yogis call "unstruck" (*anahata*), sound. Naturally we can't hear subtle sound with our everyday ears; for this we need to train our special "yogic ear" with constant meditation practice. Subtle sound is, as it were, like a homing device: when we hear it with our yogic ear, we know we're heading in the right direction and getting closer to the goal of our practice. The yogis describe subtle sound in concrete terms as being similar to that of the ocean waves, various drums, a gong, and a horn, but they also describe it in ways quite unimaginable to us. The subtle sound has been compared to the "sound of clouds," which suggests that the "unstruck" is unlike any sound we've heard before.

The yogis distinguish between four "states" (*bhava*) of sound. In effect these are four stages of world/word creation, though it might be more accurate to say that all sound, whether random or organized, issues from the same "soundless" source in three increasingly "sound-full" stages or involutes. The source itself is called the "supreme sound" or "supreme voice" (*shabda brahman* or *para vac*), similar to what we in the West call the Logos (which means both "speech, word" and "reason") or the Word of God. "In the beginning was the Word, and the Word was with God, and the Word was God." The ancient Greeks envisaged the Logos as the creative and governing spirit of the world, while for the early Christians the Word was divine wisdom incarnated in the person of Jesus.

Shabda brahman is the transcendent, perfectly quiescent background to sound, in which there's as yet no differentiation into subject and object, and so no world and nothing to say. In shabda brahman the world/word exists only in potential. But each of us is ultimately rooted in this absolute, and given the proper training, we can develop our inborn ability to tap into its creative, transformative, and emancipative power.

The first faint stirring of shabda brahman's world- (or word-) building impulse—actually the first moment of consciousness in the universe and the individual—gives rise to the second stage of sound, called "visible sound" (*pashyanti shabda*). This unusual phrase needs some explanation, since *pashyanti shabda* is still located in the subtle sphere and certainly can neither be seen by the physical eye nor heard by the physical ear. The root of this Sanskrit word means, in its simplest and most literal sense, "to see, look at, observe." Here, though, it's used in a more specific sense that means "to see with the spiritual eye, to have insight or discernment." With the world that arises at the level of second-stage sound, there's still no distinct separation between self and other, only an intense desire to be a self, an "I," and to "see" (and hear) oneself in and through the "that," the world of objects.

The third stage is called the "middle sound" (*madhyama shabda*) simply because of its location in the middle of the second and fourth states, between the sheer possibility of the world/word and the world's palpable inception and sounding out. Madhyama shabda is also known as "hidden speech" because it's associated with thought or ideation and reason. With this stage we're finally in familiar territory. Now a clear difference is established between self and other, and the Word is cut up into words, though not as yet fully "spoken" as the world/word.

Finally we arrive at the fourth stage of this involutionary scheme, "corporeal sound" (*vaikhara shabda*). Several interesting explanations have been offered for the Sanskrit word *vaikhari*: it's what is in that which is most solid (*vikhara*), the body; or it's that which certainly (*vai*) enters (*ri*) the space (*kha*) of the ear. Corporeal sound, whether random or organized, is the sound (and the only sound) known to Western science, the audible sound of the everyday world, including human speech (*vac*).

This graduated emergence of everyday sound from its soundless source has been compared to the process of human birth, in which the child first exists only as an abstraction in the loving thoughts of its parents, then as a fertilized egg, then as a fetus, and finally as a neonate. Similarly, every sound is ultimately rooted in and infused with some quality of its "parent," *shabda brahman*. Moreover every sound we make is a "child" of ours, and so a little world-creation. But only the yogis are aware of this intrinsic connection between their sounds and the soundless source. Their words then, as Vyasa remarks in his commentary to the *Yoga Sutra* (2.36), are "infallible." If a yogi "says to somebody 'Be virtuous' he becomes virtuous, if he says 'Go to heaven' he goes to heaven" (translation by Swami Hariharananda Aranya). The rest of us are unconscious of this connection; consequently our words are cut off from their source, which makes them confused and confusing, and so a source only of ignorance (*avidya*) and bondage.

>> *Could you go into* Nada Yoga, *which is described in the fourth chapter of the* Yoga Sutra?

By joining ear and thumb, they listen to the sound of the space within the heart. . . . Going beyond their separate characteristics, they meet their end in the supreme soundless unmanifest *brahman*. There they are without separate nature . . . like different flavors combined into sweetness.

Maitri Upanishad 6.22

The knowable exists inside the audible reverberation of the sound not struck. . . . The soundless is said to be the highest Brahman and the highest Atman.

Hatha Yoga Pradipika 4.100–101

While we in the West study the physical manifestations of sound, the yogis' have, through their meditation techniques, tapped into the metaphysical source of all sound, which they call the "supreme" or "Absolute sound" (*shabda brahman*) or "supreme voice" (*para vac*). There they discovered a vibratory power that shapes, pervades, and ultimately reabsorbs the whole universe.

We can't, of course, hear this source-sound, which the yogis call "unstruck" (*anahata*), with our everyday ears. Nonetheless it's the foundation of a practice called *Nada Yoga,* the Yoga of [Subtle] Sound. We don't hear much about Nada Yoga nowadays, but it's described in some detail by Svatmarama near the end of the *Hatha Yoga Pradipika.* Though the practice may seem at first glance very esoteric, he says it's suitable even for the "self-ignorant"—which is, I have a sneaking suspicion, a reference to you and me. And Svatmarama says that of the one-and-a-quarter crore of ways to liberation—a crore, in case you're wondering, equals ten million rupees—Nada Yoga is the best.

So how do we practice Nada Yoga? Pretty simple. First we have to purify our nadis, presumably with asana and pranayama. That should only take, oh, a few years. Next sit in a yoga seat and perform what Svatmarama calls Shiva's Seal, though in our terminology it's the Six Openings Seal, the one in which our thumbs block the openings to the ear canals. Finally, listen for and meditate on the subtle source-sound picked up in your *right* ear. The sound supposedly transforms the mind by "masking" or blocking out (much like white noise masks all other noises) and ultimately dissolving all its internal chatter (a spiritual version of white noise) at which point our self-identity with the actual source of the sound, Brahman, is revealed. Svatmarama illustrates this process with several vivid images. "This sharp stick of nada," he says, "can control the mind roaming in the garden of objects like a noble elephant in rut." Or, he says, "Nada is like a net that catches the deer of the mind."

The unstruck sound is apparently picked up in our body, just like a radio picks up transmissions from a station, by the "most gracious channel," the *sushumna nadi*. According to Svatmarama, as you penetrate into the subtleties of Nada Yoga, the benefits of the practice become increasingly appealing. First you experience bliss—not a bad start, but only a taste of what's to come. Next you acquire a "divine body, radiance, divine fragrance, freedom from disease, and a full heart," then freedom from "defects, misery, old age, disease, hunger, and sleep," and finally—ready?—liberation, in which you become the "maker of creation and destruction."

Naturally since the unstruck sound is subtle, it's hard to describe just what it sounds like. The yogis list several sounds to listen for, which I've listed following the section on Hatha Meditation on page 214.

In his *Stalking the Wild Pendulum* (1977), Itzhak Bentov (1923–1979) proposed what he called a "physio-kundalini" model that accounted for, among other things, these curious subtle sounds. The model is much too complex to detail here, but essentially Bentov theorized that in meditation the practitioner's brain begins to oscillate rhythmically. This pendulum-like movement generates standing waves that surround the brain, and are sent to the middle ear where they're converted into sound, and then perceived as whistling, hissing, chirping, or roaring.

>> *What is a* mantra?

Though all sound radiates out from *shabda brahman*, and possesses some degree of its power, some sounds, called *mantras*, are far more powerful than others. The yogis' science of sound is often called mantra wisdom (*mantra vidya*) or mantra teaching (*mantra shashtra*). You've likely heard the word *mantra* before, and maybe even recite mantras in your daily practice. It's a word that has no exact correlation in English. Though it's often translated as "hymn" or "prayer," these words have associations in English that are misleading when applied to mantra, and so it's probably best left untranslated.

A mantra is literally an "instrument of thought" (the Sanskrit *man* means "to think"), though not the discursive thinking most of us engage in most of the time. A more complete definition might be "an instrument of concentrated or meditative thought about the Self." Mantras are really essentially sacred formulas, through which we can invoke and affirm our identity with the soundless source, but *only* if they're properly pronounced with due attention paid to their essential meaning, and held in strictest secrecy. They can consist of a single letter, a syllable or string of syllables, a word, or a whole sentence. The building blocks of mantras are the fifty letters of the Sanskrit alphabet, the holy, "perfected" (*samskrita*) language of India. Collectively these letters or sounds are known as "divine city writing" (*deva nagari*); individually each is affectionately called a "little mother" (*matrika*) or a "seed" (*bija*)—that is, a packet of spiritual energy, an aspect or spark of *shabda brahman*.

There are more mantras than we can count. Probably the most famous mantra in the West is the monosyllable OM, the "root mantra" (*mula mantra*), which has been venerated and chanted by practitioners for thousands of years.

» *What is the "unspoken mantra"* (ajapa mantra)?

I'd like to teach you a mantra that, while surely not as well known as OM, is nevertheless on the lips of every living creature, breath after breath, throughout its life. It's called the "unspoken mantra" (*ajapa mantra*).

The yogis say that each inhale and each exhale makes a low but nonetheless distinct sound. Sit back now, close your eyes, and listen carefully for a few minutes to the sound of your everyday breathing. (Incidentally, I was once taught that the "yogic ear" is situated at the back of the skull, just in front of that little bony bump you can feel at the apex of the neck.

You might want to "listen" from this spot as an experiment.) Don't get discouraged if you can't hear the mantra right away—just pretend that you do, and eventually it will come.

The yogis say that if we listen in such a manner we will, in time, hear a hissing SA-sound with each inhale, and a breathy HA-sound with each exhale (though in some old instructional manuals the sounds are reversed). Joined together the two syllables make the mantra SAHAM (sometimes spelled SOHAM). This mantra, which we all speak with every breath we take from cradle to grave, bears witness to our eternal identity with the soundless source: "That (SA) am I (HA)." Try tuning in to the unspoken mantra for a few minutes several times each day, especially when you're feeling stressed or out of sorts. The practice will naturally draw your awareness inward, slow the speed of your breathing, and help soothe the tumultuous fluctuations (*vṛtti*) of your consciousness.

» What is the "humming" (pranava) OM?

There are said to be seventy million primary mantras, so as you can imagine, they come in all shapes and sizes. A mantra, as noted, can be one or more sentences, a single word, or even a single syllable. The longer mantras can be perfectly intelligible or mystifyingly unintelligible, at least to the uninitiated. Single-syllable mantras, which are the easiest to remember and recite, are called "seed (*bija*) mantras." The idea is that just as a tiny seed "contains" an enormous tree, so each bija "contains" a great reservoir of spiritual energy.

One of the oldest and most famous bijas is OM. Scholars speculate that thousands of years ago it originated as an interjection (something like our "Oh!") during Vedic rituals, and signified a kind of agreement or compliance: "for whenever one assents to anything he says simply 'OM'" (CU 1.1.8). Tradition also pictures OM as the male seed that fertilizes the female mantra, and so its chanting precedes any ritual recitation of scripture.

In the *Yoga Sutra*, OM is referred to as the *pranava*, literally "humming," a word that derives from *pranu*, "to reverberate." This latter word, in turn, stems from the root *nu*, "to praise or command," but also "to sound or shout." From its ritual origins, OM gradually came to be understood and heard as the audible expression of the "soundless" Brahman, the transcendental, attributeless ground of reality. In this respect, OM is the "primordial seed" (*adi bija*) of the universe—this whole world, says one old text, "is nothing but OM" (CU 2.23.3).

OM is also supposedly the source of the fifty letters of the Sanskrit alphabet. As all words are "bored through with OM" (CU 2.23.3), it's considered to be the "root mantra" (*mula mantra*) from which all other mantras emerge; as it encapsulates the essence of the many thousands of hymns in the Veda, OM is the "word which all the Vedas rehearse" (KU 2.15).

Patanjali equates OM with the "master" (*ishvara*), and teaches that by chanting it as we contemplate its meaning, our consciousness becomes "one-pointed" and fit for meditation. "Through the glory of such chanting and of such Yoga, the supreme soul is revealed" (Vyasa's commentary to YS 1.28). Lama Govinda, in a similar vein, writes that OM expresses and leads to the "experience of the infinite within us."[33]

We can also meditate on the four "measures" or parts of OM. Though commonly spelled OM, the mantra actually consists of three letters, *A, U,* and *M* (in Sanskrit, whenever an initial *A* is followed by *U,* they coalesce into *O*). Each of these three parts has numerous metaphysical associations, which themselves serve as meditative seeds. For example, *A* represents our waking state, which is also the subjective consciousness of the outer world; *U* the dreaming state, or the consciousness of our inner world of thoughts, dreams, memories, etc.; finally *M* is the dreamless state of deep sleep, when consciousness is devoid of all content.

By meditating on the meaning of each of these letters in turn, we're transported progressively through the three states of ordinary consciousness to the mantra's fourth part, the so-called after-sound (*anusvara*). OM (as is typical of bijas) ends with a kind of nasalized or vibratory sound indicated by a small dot (*bindu*) placed below the final letter and sounded like the "n" in the French *bon*. This sound-vibration slowly dissolves into silence, symbolic of the "fourth" (*chaturta* or *turiya*) or transcendent state of consciousness, equated with Brahman. It's described as the "acme" or crown of the mantra, which is "tranquil, soundless, fearless, sorrowless, blissful, satisfied, steadfast, immovable, immortal, unshaken, enduring" (MU 6.23).

» *Why isn't there any meditation in Hatha Yoga?*

If we pick up just about any popular Hatha Yoga instructional manual published in this country since 1950, we will typically find a healthy dose of asana, maybe a smattering of pranayama, and not much else. Take as examples the two highly influential books by B. K. S. Iyengar, *Light on Yoga* (1966) and its follow-up, *Light on Pranayama* (1981). Of the 340-odd pages in the former, 173 are dedicated to asana, and 23 to pranayama. And meditation? Well, even though Iyengar emphatically insists he's teaching authentic Classical Yoga, which is, as we have seen, nothing but an intense form of meditation, he devotes less than two pages to the topic in *Light on Yoga* (along with a photo of himself sitting in *dhyana*). *Light on Pranayama* tells much the same tale. Of its nearly three hundred pages, one hundred apply to pranayama, nine to meditation. The idea that yoga is a physical endeavor is largely accurate so far as modern yoga is concerned (though many yoga teachers are now beginning to integrate meditation into their teaching), but it is certainly not true about traditional Hatha Yoga practice.

Proof? We can find it as far back as the eleventh century C.E., in the oldest book of the Hatha Yoga canon, the *Kaula Jnana Nirnaya*, traditionally attributed to Matsyendra. The book's teaching is presented as a dialogue between Shiva, called Bhairava ("frightful, formidable"), and his spouse, Devi, "goddess." Devi grills Shiva about all aspects of yoga, such as the acquisition of supernormal powers, the conquest of death and the secret of long life, the nature of the Self, and of course, final emancipation. Shiva replies, more often than not, by giving instructions on how and where to meditate. Indeed, much of the fourteenth chapter, for example, is devoted to meditation, including meditative practices on the cakras, the *brahma* knot (*granthi*), a light above the head, the heart, the throat, and the center of the forehead, and fissures of the skull.

Closer to our own time, we can turn to the *Shiva Samhita* (which is much easier to find a copy of than the *Kaula Jnana Nirnaya*). Here, in the fifth chapter, we encounter detailed descriptions of eight different meditation exercises. Among these are:

Meditation on the Image in the Sky (5.29–35). In this meditation the yogi begins by staring at his own shadow on a sunny day, then quickly turns his gaze to the sky, re-creating there the image of himself. With this practice he might expect, among other benefits, long life, the ability to travel through the air, and liberation.

Meditation on the Inner Light and Subtle Sounds (5.36–46). With his fingers, the yogi blocks the openings of his head—the ears, eyes, nose, and mouth—and meditates on the inner light (research reveals this is a phenomenon known as "entoptic," which means "occurring inside the eye," caused by the pressure of the fingers on the retina). Eventually he becomes absorbed in Brahman and reaches nirvana.

Then if he listens to the subtle sounds, which sound like a swarm of bees, a bell, or thunder, he becomes absorbed in the "ether of consciousness" (*cid askasha*) (of course, since the sounds are subtle and not actual, the words used to describe them are conveniences; this means, for example, that there's one subtle sound that, if we had to characterize it in a way a non-yogi could understand, we'd say it sounded like a flute).

Meditation on the Well of the Throat (*Kantha Kupa*, 5.61–62). By focusing his attention at the jugular notch, what yogis call "the well of the throat," the yogi attains the "supreme state" (*paramam padam*), even if he's a bad person.

Meditation on the Tip of the Nose (6.68–69). By focusing his attention here, the yogi becomes an "aerial being" (*khecara*, "moving in the air").

Meditation on the Back of the Head (6.71). By focusing his attention here, the yogi conquers death.

THINK OF NOTHING

There should be no thought of the external, nor any thought within. Excluding all thought he [the yogi] should think of nothing.

SVATMARAMA, *Hatha Yoga Pradipika* 4.57

Abandoning all selfish desires born of his own selfish will, a man should learn to restrain his unruly senses with his mind. Gradually he becomes calm and controls his understanding; focusing on the Self, he should think of nothing at all.

Bhagavad Gita 6.25

I'm trying to think but nothing happens.

CURLY HOWARD

The scene: Stan and Ollie have joined the French Foreign Legion, so that Ollie can forget a failed love affair with a Parisian beauty. Out in the desert, they're assigned to laundry duty, and it isn't going well. Stan is making his usual fine mess of things . . .

OLLIE. Haven't I got enough trouble without you making it tougher?

STAN. Well, it's your own fault. If you hadn't fallen in love with Georgette we wouldn't be here.

OLLIE. Will you stop reminding me of that! Here I am trying to forget, and you keep talking about it all the time. Now here's another day wasted.

STAN. Well, maybe you don't try hard enough. If you can't forget, why don't you try and *pretend* to forget?

OLLIE. How can anybody *pretend* to forget?

STAN. Well, I know if it was me, I'd sit down and relax, I'd close my eyes, and I'd concentrate and I'd think of nothing. Wouldn't be long then, that's what I'd do.

OLLIE. Say, I think you've got something there.

STAN. I know I've got something. Why don't you take a whirl at it?

Ollie sits down, supports his chin in his hands, and closes his eyes.

STAN. Now don't think of anything.

OLLIE. I won't.

From the film The Flying Deuces (1939),
starring Stan Laurel and Oliver Hardy

The origin of Hatha Yoga (Version 3)

Once upon a time, on the bank of a river, a fisherman happened upon some wandering ascetics engaged in their secret rites of yoga. His curiosity aroused, he put aside his net and boldly greeted them, asking what they were doing. The ascetics, who hadn't noticed the fisherman's presence, were horrified. As many of the old books caution, yoga knowledge is only potent (*virya*) when concealed; if carelessly revealed to the uninitiated, it's rendered totally impotent (*nirvirya*, see, e.g., YS 1.11). What made the situation worse, however, was that the outsider was low caste, and earned his daily bread by killing living creatures, a grievous sin to the ascetics. But after they spoke with the fisherman for a while, they found him to be as innocent as a child and worthy of their trust, and so they opened up to him. They praised their yogic way of life, learned from the god Shiva, and described how it led to both self-liberation and the acquisition of "supernormal powers" (*siddhi*). They warned the fisherman that if he told anyone about this encounter and what they'd said, the great goddess, Parvati, Shiva's spouse, would surely destroy him.

The fisherman might not have been worldly wise, but he was no fool, and so he promised to keep the ascetics' secrets to himself. But their words had roused some deep yearning in his soul, and with hands pressed in *anjali mudra* he humbly begged them for admittance into their fold. Realizing he was truly a "qualified aspirant" (*adhikarin*), the leader of the ascetics duly initiated the fisherman and taught him about yoga. As they were leaving, the ascetics assured him that if he practiced diligently, he soon would gain immortality and enormous power.

The fisherman immediately abandoned his familiar everyday world and, as legend has it, retired to a hermitage on Sandwip Island in the Bay of Bengal (just off the coast of present-day Bangladesh). For the next six months he wholeheartedly devoted himself to yoga. Then one day, while taking his daily bath at the river, in a bizarrely ironic turn of events, he was attacked and swallowed by a gigantic marine animal. The story doesn't say exactly what the animal was; its name, aptly enough, is the "seizer" (*graha*), which might indicate a demon of some kind or a crocodile. Whatever it was, it was huge, as large as a mountain, with a body that shone with an otherworldly light. After seizing the man, it swam off, with the ex-fisherman still very much alive in its belly.

At this point, two new characters enter the story, the husband-and-wife deities Shiva and Parvati ("Mountain"). It seems that Parvati had asked her husband to instruct her in the secrets of yoga, and so, to avoid prying ears, the pair made their way to an uninhabited island far out at sea. As Shiva began his teaching, the immense animal with the human cargo in its belly swam up to shore, close enough so that the fisherman managed to hear the god's words. Now Shiva's words weren't like yours or mine—ordinary words that may or may not have an impact on the listener. Rather, he spoke with the force of utter truthfulness (*satya*), and when this is the case, as Vyasa comments on *Yoga Sutra* 2.36, such words become "unfailingly efficacious." By listening to and absorbing Shiva's teaching on self-liberation, the ex-fisherman became liberated.

>> *You often talk in class about the differences between "traditional Hatha Yoga" and "modern Hatha Yoga." Could you put all your thoughts down in one place, please?*

Let's start with traditional Hatha Yoga. Here are some of its essential characteristics:

Gender: Unlike today, when most yoga practitioners are female, traditional Hatha Yoga was the province mostly of male renunciates, though there is evidence that in later years householders and women were admitted into the fold (albeit as second-class citizens).

Initiation: There were no books to buy, nor public classes to attend; the only way to learn the practice was to be initiated by a Self-realized teacher or guru, and this was apparently very hard to achieve. The initiation is a reenactment of the original Hatha Yoga teaching, in which the deity (usually Shiva) passes on the knowledge of the practice to the first human teacher (usually Matsyendra). We have seen some examples of the enormous efforts undertaken by hopeful practitioners to win a guru's attention and trust. (See Chapter 1 and the story of King Brihadratha and the sage Shakayanya.)

Appearance: The behavior and appearance of yogis was bizarre, purposely calculated to set them apart from the "straight" world. They often went naked, covered their bodies with ashes, and/or carried a skull as a begging bowl. Such practices placed them on the very fringes of society. (Note, however, that Svatmarama declares in *Hatha Yoga Pradipika* 1.66 that success isn't achieved by "wearing the right clothes.")

Behavior: The yogis didn't have much interest in conforming to socially acceptable behavior, since presumably they had little to do with the outside world. Only some translations of the *Hatha Yoga Pradipika* include mention of the yamas and niyamas, the Classical behavioral guidelines that regulate our relations with others, and the way we conduct our personal lives. Other versions exclude the yamas and niyamas entirely. (Later commentators have explained this omission by saying that these would already have been well known to yogis.)

Practice: Practice dominated daily life. A yogi practiced at least three or four (or even five) times a day (HYP 2.11) at the "junctions," *samdhya* (dawn, noon, sunset, midnight). For example, Svatmarama, commenting on the three "greats" (*maha mudra, maha bandha, maha vedha*), says "they are to be done eight times every day" (HYP 3.31), which means every three hours. *Viparita karani mudra* (usually interpreted to mean Shoulder Stand, though sometimes practiced as Head Stand) is ideally practiced for "three hours every day" (HYP 3.82). Practice was tailored to suit the individual student. Each student was viewed as a unique individual with varying strengths and weaknesses, so that the structure and timing of the practice had to be adjusted to account for the student's capacities.

Secrecy: Like the Veda before it, the teaching on Hatha Yoga was thought to have a divine origin, the deity Shiva (see the three versions of the "origin of Hatha Yoga" in this chapter). Consequently, in the minds of the yogis, that teaching and the practices that embodied it were imbued with Shiva's superhuman power. The practices then were the means whereby they could tap into that power, and become almost god-like themselves. Obviously, such power could be disastrously misused if somehow developed by the wrong person.

Like the teaching of the Veda, that of Hatha Yoga was kept top secret and reserved strictly for students who had been duly initiated by a Self-realized guru. Non-initiates, no doubt the great majority of the Indian population, were denied any and all access to the teachings.

But this wasn't the only reason the teaching was kept secret. If we want to use a river as a source of power, we might build a dam across it. This stops the rivers's flow, and the reservoir that collects behind the dam is essentially a store of potential energy. In the same way, a yogi is advised to keep her practice a secret (*gupta*). This serves to "dam up" the energy generated by her practice and provide a vast reservoir of transformative power. Gheranda warns us that the practice becomes "impotent" (*nirvirya*) if it's revealed (GS 1.11).

Today, of course, the written records of these secret teachings that once were reserved exclusively for the "in crowd," and that promised perfect health and long life, extraordinary powers beyond our wildest dreams, and release from the trammels of ego dominance, are now easily purchased by anyone on Amazon for a few dollars. The question is: are these formerly hush-hush teachings still potent and possibly dangerous? And the answer is, of course, as it so often is with yoga questions: it all depends.

By themselves the books do contain some useful information that we can apply to our practice. But at the same time, by themselves, they're probably not enough to get us over the top on Self-realization or help us develop superhuman powers in order to rule the world. For that we'll need a Self-realized guru; as Gheranda reminds us: *samadhi* is achieved by those who are devoted to their guru and fortunate (*bhagya*, "lucky") enough to merit his compassion (*krpa*) and grace (*prasasda*) (GS 7.1).[34]

Now for modern Hatha Yoga.

Behavior: The practice had to be "tamed" and "moralized"—no more running around naked, smeared with ashes, acting crazy. Whether or not traditional Hatha Yoga had behavioral guidelines, modern Hatha Yoga needs them. The vast majority of yoga practitioners today are householders, and if it is to be efficacious our practice surely must help guide our actions in the complex, workaday world in which we all live.

We can take the yamas and niyamas of Classical Yoga as our foundation for ethical action, and adopt others that seem useful (as long as we apply them only to ourselves and don't impose our idealized standards on anyone else). We might start with the injunctions that are included in Hatha Yoga texts but which are missing in Classical Yoga. The yamas here include kindliness (*daya*), equanimity (*arjava*), patience (*kshama*), firmness of mind (*dhriti*), and proper diet (*mitahara*). As for the niyamas: giving alms to those in need (*dana*).

Powers: The acquisition and intensification of power—one of the goals of traditional yoga—has been downplayed or even denied in modern Hatha Yoga, for without a personal guide such power could easily be misused or abused, and the pursuit of *siddhis* could lead a student down a disastrous path of self-aggrandizement.

Practice: The time needed to perform the practice has had to be decreased, radically so, to accommodate the demands of modern life. Instead of three or four (or even five) substantial practices daily we now get ten- or fifteen-minute exercise "quickies" squeezed into our day when the opportunity arises. Practice, once tailored by the teacher to suit the individual, has of necessity been standardized. Students are now instructed en masse by teachers who may know nothing more about them than their first names, if that, and all receive essentially the same instructions regardless of experience or capacity.

Because the practice times are shortened, it's common now for the teacher to telescope one practice into another so that one exercise does double duty. So, for example, the teacher may instruct the students in her class to choose a yama, let's say non-harming (*ahimsa*), and express it through an asana. This surely is an interesting exercise that challenges the extent of the students' understanding of both the pose and *ahimsa*, though of course it completely revamps the original intent of both exercises.

» Why do we say "namaste" at the end of a yoga class? What does it mean?

Namaste comes from the word *namas,* which means to "bow to, to salute reverentially, to adore," along with the pronoun *te,* "you." Literally then, *namaste* means "I bow to you." To be accurate, since *te* is singular, the word should only be used when saluting one person. What this means in a yoga class is that the students, who are acknowledging the teacher, should say *namaste*. But the teacher responding to a roomful of people (or at least more than two) should ideally use the plural form of "you" (*vaha*): *namo vaha* (nuh-mo-vuh-huh).

Namaste is usually accompanied with a hand gesture or mudra called *anjali mudra*. In fact, this mudra is so closely associated with the expression of namaste that it's not unusual to hear novice teachers, when preparing for the salutation, say something like, "Bring your hands into namaste." Also be aware that the hands are positioned according to whom you're saluting. For the teacher the hands are brought opposite the sternum, before the face for a respected elder, and above the head for a deity.

Namaste, by the way, is often interpreted to mean "The divine in me bows to the divine in you." This is no doubt a beautiful sentiment, but Indian acquaintances of mine inform me this is a bit overdone, and that "namaste" is no more than a token of respect.

» *You once mentioned that the old yogis had three goals in mind for their practice. Could you discuss them again?*

1. The first goal was Self-realization, which is more or less the goal of all yoga schools.
2. The second goal was long life, which was sought for two reasons. Since the practice was so time-consuming, the yogis wanted to give themselves more years to practice and reach their goals. Moreover, once their goals were achieved, the Hatha yogis, unlike some of their opposite numbers in other yoga schools, wanted to remain embodied and enjoy this beautiful world as much as they could. This is known as "living liberation" (*jivan mukti*). Svatmarama lists a lineage of adepts who have broken the punishing "rod of time" (*kala danda*), and wander freely through "Brahma's egg," the universe.
3. The third goal was power. As I mentioned, modern Hatha Yoga tends to downplay this aspect of traditional Hatha Yoga, fearing two consequences: that mainstream, middle-class Westerners will be turned off by reports of strange and superhuman powers (and

take up tai chi instead of yoga); and that such reports will, on the other hand, attract Darth Vader wannabes, who pursue yoga for all the wrong reasons (you might refer back to the question on the powers [*siddhi*] in Chapter 4 and the quote from David Lorenzen).

» *I want to study the literature of traditional Hatha Yoga. What primary books should I read?*

The literature of Hatha Yoga is far more extensive than we might imagine. I recently compiled a Hatha Yoga bibliography that totals about seventy books, and I suspect there are at least that many again that can be added to the roster. But the majority of these texts haven't been translated into English, or if they have, they aren't readily available at your corner bookstore or even online.

Anyway, to be honest, most Hatha Yoga books that have been translated into English and are more or less readily available aren't especially gripping reads. Their philosophy, as Gerald Larson points out, amounts to either a "simplified, monistic Vedanta," or an "equally simplified version of Shaiva and/or Shakti theology."[35] The authors/compilers were mainly interested in practical matters, "ritualistic manipulation of the body's postures . . . fluids and . . . breathing mechanisms for the sake of attaining enhanced physical strength, greater mental clarity and altered states of awareness of various kinds."[36] But before you rush out to buy one of these books, hoping you'll learn the secrets for acquiring these highly desirable qualities, understand that they weren't written originally as instructional manuals for a mass audience of nonspecialists. Much like the *Yoga Sutra* (see Chapter 4), the texts typically provide just a brief outline of the practice; the details were supposed to be filled in directly by the guru. As a result, the terse instructions in these texts are mostly too obscure or ambiguous to be of much use as practical guides.

Still many of the books do have some interest for anyone seriously studying the history of Hatha Yoga, and it is possible to pick up a few ideas about what the traditional practices were and what they might have been like. So if you're determined to read primary texts, you should start with the *Hatha Yoga Pradipika*, the mid-fifteenth-century text compiled by Svatmarama Yogendra. The *Hatha Yoga Pradipika* is a book of firsts. Among them, according to scholar James Mallinson, the text is the first to identify four practices that would lay the practical foundation for subsequent Hatha texts; these four are *asana, pranayama* (or *kumbhaka*), *mudra* (which includes *bandha*), and concentration on the subtle inner sound (*nada anu sandhana*).

Along with the *Hatha Yoga Pradipika*, two other primary books are popular and thus easy to acquire. The *Gheranda Samhita* and the *Shiva Samhita* are both "compendiums" (*samhita*), which have been expertly translated by Mallinson. The *Gheranda Samhita*, a seventeenth-century text, is much like the *Hatha Yoga Pradipika*: short on philosophy, long on practice. In fact, it addresses practice in much greater detail than does the *Hatha Yoga Pradipika*. Though about seventy verses shorter in length, it teaches far more asanas (thirty-two to the *Hatha Yoga Pradipika*'s fifteen) and mudras (twenty-five versus ten). The *Shiva Samhita* is the odd bird of the three. Most commentators make it contemporary with the *Gheranda Samhita*, though Mallinson dates it to the fifteenth century. What's odd about it, though, is that, unlike its two companions, it's fairly heavy on philosophy, at least on matters regarding the subtle body. But even so, a good three-quarters of its 640 verses are dedicated in some way to practice. The longest chapter by far, consuming about forty percent of the text, is the last, the fifth, which concerns meditation.

There are maybe a dozen other books a serious student may want to look through. They are listed in the back matter in chronological order, from the earliest to the most recent.

Notes

CHAPTER 1

1. Edwin Bryant, trans., *The Yoga Sutras of Patanjali* (New York: Northpoint Press, 2009), 5.

2. Usharbudh Arya, trans., *Yoga-Sutras of Patanjali: With the Exposition of Vyasa,* vol. 1, *Samadhi-pada* (Honesdale, PA: Himalayan International Institute of Yoga Science and Philosophy of the U.S.A., 1986), 63.

3. Romesh Dutt, *A History of Civilization in Ancient India* (Calcutta: Thacker, Spink, and Co., 1889), 302.

4. Harold Coward, *Jung and Eastern Thought* (Albany, NY: State University of New York, 1985), 10.

5. Carl Jung, quoted in Harry Old Meadow, *Journeys East: 20th Century Western Encounters with Eastern Religious Traditions* (Bloomington, IN: World Wisdom, 2004), 100.

6. Carl Jung and Richard Wilhelm, *The Secret of the Golden Flower: A Chinese Book of Life* (New York: Mariner Books, 1962), 89.

7. Georg Feuerstein, *Tantra: The Path of Ecstasy* (Boston: Shambhala, 1998), 283.

8. Margaret and James Stutley, "Brahmana," *Harper's Dictionary of Hinduism* (New York: Harper & Row, 1977), 51.

9. Gerald James Larson and Ram Shankar Bhattacharya, eds., *Encyclopedia of Indian Philosophies,* vol. 12, *Yoga: India's Philosophy of Meditation* (Delhi: Motilal Banarsidass Publishers, 2008), 28–29.

10. Bryant, *The Yoga Sutras of Patanjali,* 5–6.

11. Georg Feuerstein, *The Deeper Dimension of Yoga: Theory and Practice* (Boston: Shambhala, 2003), 27.

12. Charles Masson, *Narrative of Various Journeys in Balochistan, Afghanistan, the Panjab, and Kalat,* vol. 1 (London: Richard Bentley, 1844), 453.

13. John Roach, "Faceless Indus Valley City Puzzles Archaeologists," *National Geographic*, http://science.nationalgeographic.com/science/archaeology /mohenjo-daro/

14. Gavin Flood, *An Introduction to Hinduism* (Cambridge: Cambridge University Press, 1996), 28–29.

15. David Gordon White, *Sinister Yogis* (Chicago: University of Chicago Press, 2009), 49, 81.

16. Arya, *Yoga-Sutras of Patanjali*, 70.

17. Georg Feuerstein, *The Yoga-Sutra of Patanjali* (Rochester, VT: Inner Traditions International, 1989), 59.

18. Bryant, *The Yoga Sutras of Patanjali*, 6.

19. Mircea Eliade, *Yoga: Immortality and Freedom* (Princeton, NJ: Princeton University Press, 1969), 7.

20. Bryant, *The Yoga Sutras of Patanjali*, 251.

21. Georg Feuerstein, "Nyaya," *The Encyclopedia of Yoga and Tantra* (Boston: Shambhala, 2011), 251.

22. Ibid., 388.

23. John Dowson, *A Classical Dictionary of Hindu Mythology* (London: Routledge & Kegan Paul, 1972), 294.

24. Karlfried Graf Durkheim, *The Call for the Master* (New York: E.P. Dutton, 1989), 19.

25. Ibid., 5.

26. Ibid., 39.

27. Ibid., 34.

28. Ibid., 54.

29. Ibid., 58.

30. Ibid., 59.

31. Ibid., 63.

CHAPTER 2

1. Henry Yule and A. C. Burrell, *Hobson-Jobson: The Anglo-Indian Dictionary* (Herfordshire, UK: Wordsworth Reference, 1996), 792.

2. Frederick Bodmer, *The Loom of Language* (New York: W.W. Norton, 1972), 411.

3. William Whitney, *Sanskrit Grammar* (Cambridge, MA: Harvard University Press, 1973), 1.

4. Wendy Doniger, *The Hindus* (New York: Penguin Press, 2009), 5.

5. Max Müller, *A Sanskrit Grammar* (New Delhi: Asian Publication Services, 1975), 4.

6. Sampad and Vijay, *The Wonder That Is Sanskrit* (Ahmedabad, India: Mapin Publishing, 2002), 111.

7. Atma Institute, owned by Bhaktivedanta Society. www.atmainstitute.org/sanskrit.htm.

8. "The Vedic Foundation: Valuable Resources," compiled from *The True History and the Religion of India,* by Swami Prakasha Saraswati. www.thevedic foundation.org/valuable_resources/Sanskrit-The_Mother_of_All _Languages_partI.htm.

9. "Encyclopedia of Authentic Hinduism," compiled from *The True History and the Religion of India,* by Swami Prakasha Saraswati. www.encylopediaof authentichindism.org/index.html.

10. Sheldon Pollock, "The Death of Sanskrit," *Comparative Studies in Society and History, International Quarterly* 43.2 (April 2001), 392–425.

11. Vasudha Narayanan, *The Vernacular Veda: Revalation, Recitation, and Ritual* (Columbia, SC: University of South Carolina Press, 1994), 49.

12. A. L. Basham, *The Wonder That Was India* (New York: Grove Press, 1959), 388.

13. Dowson, *A Classical Dictionary of Hindu Mythology,* 228.

14. Sampad and Vijay, *The Wonder That Is Sanskrit,* 147.

15. Robert Goldman and Sally Goldman, *Devavanipraveshika: An Introduction to the Sanskrit Language* (Berkeley, CA: Center for South Asian Studies, 2002), xii.

16. Müller, *A Sanskrit Grammar,* 3.

17. Arthur Macdonell, *A Sanskrit Grammar for Students* (London: Oxford University Press, 1975), 2.

18. Benjamin Walker, "Nagari," *The Hindu World: An Encyclopedic Survey of Hinduism* (New York: Frederick A. Praeger, 1968), 108.

19. Walter Maurer, *The Sanskrit Language* (London: Routledge, 2009), 13.

20. Michael Coulson, *Complete Sanskrit* (Chicago: Contemporary Books, 1992), 41.

21. Maurer, *The Sanskrit Language,* 14.

22. Ibid., 20.

23. Ibid., 24.

24. Whitney, *Sanskrit Grammar,* 37.

25. Maurer, *The Sanskrit Language,* 33.

26. Ibid., 43.

CHAPTER 3

1. Maurice Bloomfield, *The Religion of the Veda* (New Delhi: Indological Book House, 1972), 41.

2. *Hymns of the Rig Veda,* translated by Ralph T. H. Griffith, Sanskrit Web, sponsor Ulrich Stiehl (accessed January 2005). http://www.sanskritweb.net /rigveda/griffith.pdf.

3. Judith Tyberg, *The Languge of the Gods* (Los Angeles: East-West Cultural Center, 1970), 87.
4. Sri Aurobindo, *The Secret of the Veda* (Pondicherry, India: Sri Aurobindo Ashram, 1987), 3.
5. Maurice Winternitz, *History of Indian Literature* (Calcutta: University of Calcutta, 1927), 187.
6. Ibid., 231.
7. Ibid., 233.
8. S. Radhakrishnan, *The Principal Upanishads* (New Delhi: Indus, 1995), 49.
9. Winternitz, *History of Indian Literature*, 233.
10. Ibid., 167.
11. Arthur Keith, *The Religion and Philosophy of the Veda and Upanishads*, part 1 (New Delhi: Motilal Banarsidass, 1989), 489.
12. Available online at www.scribd.com/doc/21724974/History-Text-and -Context-of-the-Yoga-Upanishads.
13. Jeffrey Ruff, "History, Text, and Context of the Yoga Upanishads" (PhD dissertation, 2002), 45–46.
14. Patrick Olivelle, trans., *Upanishads* (Oxford: Oxford University Press, 1996), lii n28.
15. Louis Renou, *Religions of Ancient India* (New York: Schocken Books, 1970), 18.
16. Ibid., 183.
17. Paul Deussen, *The Philosophy of the Upanishads* (New York: Dover, 1966), 13.
18. Winternitz, *History of Indian Literature*, 237 n4; Valerie Roebuck, *The Upanishads* (New Delhi: Penguin Books, 2000), 370; S. Radhakrishnan, *The Principal Upanishads*, 669; Walker, *The Hindu World*, 534; V. M. Bedekar and G. B. Palsule, *Sixty Upanishads of the Veda*, trans. by Paul Deussen, vol. 2 (Delhi: Motilal Banarsidass, 1980), 569; Olivelle, *Upanishads,* 266.
19. M. Hiriyanna, *Outlines of Indian Philosophy* (London: George Allen & Unwin, 1970), 14.
20. Ibid., 183.

CHAPTER 4

1. Surendranath Dasgupta, *A History of Indian Philosophy*, vol. 1 (New Delhi: Motilal Banarsidass, 1992), 62.
2. Winternitz, *History of Indian Literature*, 30.
3. Arya, *Yoga-Sutras of Patanjali*, 60.
4. Georg Feuerstein, *The Encyclopedia of Yoga and Tantra* (Boston: Shambhala, 2011), 201.
5. Bryant, *The Yoga Sutras of Patanjali*, xxxii.

6. Ibid., xxxii.
7. Feuerstein, *The Yoga-Sutra of Patanjali*, 59.
8. Alain Danielou, *The Gods of India* (New York: Inner Traditions, 1985), 365.
9. David Gordon White, *The Yoga Sutra of Patanjali: A Biography* (Princeton, NJ: Princeton University Press, 2014), 227.
10. Rammurti Mishra, *Yoga Sutras* (Garden City, NY: Anchor Books), 274.
11. M. N. Dvivedi, *The Yoga-Sutras of Patanjali* (New Delhi: Sri Satguru Publications, 1983), 57.
12. Feuerstein, *The Yoga-Sutra of Patanjali*, 87.
13. Walter Kaelber, *Tapta Marga: Asceticism and Initiation in Vedic India* (Albany: State University of New York, 1989), 2.
14. Ibid., 3.
15. Feuerstein, *The Yoga-Sutra of Patanjali*, 60.
16. Eliade, *Yoga: Immortality and Freedom*, 74.
17. Georg Feuerstein, *The Philosophy of Classical Yoga* (Rochester, VT: Inner Traditions International, 1996), 12.
18. George Briggs, *Gorakhnath and the Kanphata Yogis* (Delhi: Motilal Banarsidass, 1989), 270.
19. Larson and Bhattacharya, *Encyclopedia of Indian Philosophies*, 129.
20. B. K. S. Iyengar, *The Tree of Yoga* (Boston: Shambhala, 1989), 122.
21. David Lorenzen, *The Kapalikas and Kalamukhas* (Berkeley: University of California Press, 1972), 93–94.
22. Arthur Koestler, *The Lotus and the Robot* (New York: Macmillan Company, 1961), 110–11.
23. Charles Johnston, *The Yoga Sutras of Patanjali* (London: Stuart & Watkins, 1970), 7.
24. Ibid., 8–9.
25. Ibid., 95.

CHAPTER 5

1. Iyengar, *The Tree of Yoga*, 3.
2. Swami Vivekananda, *Raja Yoga* (New York: Ramakrishna-Vivekananda Center, 1982), 23.
3. Yogi Hari, *Hatha Yoga Pradipika* (Miramar, FL: Nada Productions, 2005), 204.
4. Feuerstein, *Tantra*, 53.
5. Arthur Avalon [John Woodroffe], *Shakti and Shakta* (New York: Dover, 1978), 685.
6. Joseph Campbell, *The Masks of God: Oriental Mythology* (New York: Viking Press, 1962), 200.
7. Yogi Hari, *Hatha Yoga Pradipika*, 149–50.

8. Stephan A. Hoeller, *The Gnostic Jung and the Seven Sermons to the Dead* (Wheaton, IL: Theosophical Publishing House, 1982), 159.

9. Paramahamsa Yogananda, *The Bhagavad Gita* (Los Angeles: Self-Realization Fellowship, 1995), 604.

10. Danielou, *The Gods of India*, 129.

11. Rudra Shivananda, *Being Bliss Now*, website of the Fellowship of Higher Consciousness. www.rudrashivananda.com.

12. Rai Bahadur Srira Chandra Vidyarnava, *The Daily Practice of the Hindus* (New Delhi: Oriental Books Reprint Corporation, 1979), 120.

13. Ibid., 93.

14. Dolf Hartsuiker, *Sadhus: Holy Men of India* (London: Thames & Hudson, 1993), 87.

15. Stuart Sovatsky, *Words from the Soul: Time, East/West Spirituality, and Psychotherapeutic Narrative* (Albany: State University of New York, 1998), 154.

16. M. L. Gharote and G. K. Pai, *Siddha-Siddhanta-Paddhatih* (Lonavla, India: Lonavla Yoga Institute, 2010), 167.

17. Surendranath Dasgupta, *Obscure Religious Cults* (Calcutta: Firma KLM Private Limited, 1995), 204.

18. Gudrun Bühnemann, *Eighty-four Asanas in Yoga* (New Delhi: D.K. Printworld, 2011), 27.

19. Matthew Kapstein, "King Kuñji's Banquet," in *Tantra in Practice*, ed. David Gordon White (Princeton, NJ: Princeton University Press, 2000), 52–71.

20. Danielou, *The Gods of India*, 160.

21. Arthur Avalon [John Woodroffe], *The Serpent Power* (New York: Dover, 1974), 204 n1.

22. Mark Singleton, *Yoga Body: The Origins of Modern Posture Practice* (Oxford: Oxford University Press, 2010), 221–22 n4.

23. Ibid., 14.

24. Ibid., 124.

25. Shrimant Balasahib Pandit Pratinidhi, *The Ten-Point Way to Health* (London: J. M. Dent and Sons, 1938), 24.

26. Ibid., 78.

27. Joseph Alter, *The Wrestler's Body* (New Delhi: Munshiram Manoharlal, 1997), 98.

28. Shri Yogendra, *Yoga Asanas Simplified* (Mumbai, India: Yogendra Publications Fund, 2000), 99.

29. Ibid., 100.

30. Rajah of Aundh, *The Ten Point Way to Health*, 89.

31. B. K. S. Iyengar, *Yoga Wisdom & Practice* (London: Dorling Kindersley, 2000), 34.

32. Vimla Murty and Kalyani Namjoshi, "Use of Props: An Interview with Gurji," in *70 Glorious Years of Yogacharya B. K. S. Iyengar*, edited by Geeta Iyengar (Bombay: Light on Yoga Research Trust, 1990), 395.

33. Lama Anagarika Govinda, *Foundations of Tibetan Mysticism* (New York: Samuel Weiser, 1974), 24.

34. This paragraph was inspired by a personal communication with Mark Singleton, May 9, 2016.

35. Larson and Bhattacharya, *Encyclopedia of Indian Philosophies*, 435.

36. Ibid.

Resources

CHAPTER 1

Want to Know More About the Guru?

Dürckheim, Karlfried Graf. *The Call for the Master.* New York: E. P. Dutton, 1986.

Godman, David. "The Guru." In *Be As You Are: The Teachings of Sri Ramana Maharhi,* edited by David Godman. New York: Penguin Books, 1992.

Isherwood, Christopher. *My Guru and His Disciple.* New York: Penguin Books, 1981.

Vyasa, Shri. *Guru Gita.* Pond Eddy, NY: Swami Tirth Ashram, 2006.

Want to Know More About Yoga?

Calasso, Roberto. *Ka: Stories of the Mind and Gods of India.* New York: Alfred Knopf, 1998.

Connolly, Peter. *A Student's Guide to the History and Philosophy of Yoga.* Oakville, CT: DBBC, 2007.

Feuerstein, Georg. *The Deeper Dimension of Yoga.* Boston: Shambhala, 2003.

———. *The Encyclopedia of Tantra and Yoga.* Boston: Shambhala, 2011

———. *The Path of Yoga.* Boston: Shambhala, 2011.

———. *The Yoga Tradition.* Prescott, AZ: Hohm Press, 1998.

Frawley, David. *Yoga: The Greater Tradition.* San Rafael, CA: Mandala Publishing, 2008.

Iyengar, B. K. S. *The Tree of Yoga.* Boston: Shambhala, 1989.

Samuel, Geoffrey. *The Origins of Yoga and Tantra.* Cambridge: Cambridge University Press, 2008.

Stone, Michael. *The Inner Tradition of Yoga.* Boston: Shambhala, 2008.

CHAPTER 2

Want to Know More About Sanskrit?

> There is a sense in which any translation from Sanskrit into English will remain imperfect, since many Sanskrit terms are multivalent, and their inherent meanings are piled one upon another. . . . It is not so much the case that a line of Sanskrit may have one dominant signification and several auxiliary ones, as that several significations may be present simultaneously. This fact makes it virtually impossible to capture the whole meaning of a Sanskrit sentence in a single line of English.
>
> MIKEL BURLEY, *Hatha-Yoga: Its Context, Theory, and Practice*, p. 12

After reading this rather discouraging remark about the inherent difficulty of rendering Sanskrit successfully into English, you might well ask the question: Why bother to learn Sanskrit? Why indeed. I can think of two good reasons: (1) despite my grouching about its complexity, Sanskrit is what we might call a "brain workout," guaranteed to make you think; (2) if you're a yoga geek or nerd or just a serious student, knowing even a bit of Sanskrit can open doors to new insights in the old Sanskrit yoga texts.

At last count I have fifteen Sanskrit primers in my library. Each time I bought one, I hoped it would be *the one* that would finally let me in on the secret of how to learn Sanskrit. Instead, I discovered that each has its own strengths and weaknesses, though perhaps you will find *your one* among them. I sincerely hope so. Here are the primers I recommend, in order of preference:

Egenes, Thomas. *Introduction to Sanskrit*. 2 vols. Delhi: Motilal Banarsidass, 1994.
Maurer, Walter. *The Sanskrit Language*. London: Routledge, 2009.
Goldman, Robert, and Sally Sutherland Goldman. *An Introduction to the Sanskrit Language (Devavanipraveshika)*. Berkeley: UC Berkeley Center for South Asia Studies, 2002.
Coulson, Michael. *Complete Sanskrit*. Chicago: Contemporary Books, 2010.

CHAPTER 3

Want to Know More About the Veda?

Frawley, David. *Wisdom of the Ancient Seers: Mantras of the Rig Veda*. Salt Lake City, UT: Passage Press, 1992.
The Rig Veda. Translation by Wendy Doniger. New York: Penguin Books, 1984.

Want to Know More About the Yoga Upanishads?

The Yoga-Upanishads. Translated by T. R. Srinivasa Ayyangar. Madras: Vasanta Press, 1938. http://archive.org/details/TheYogaUpanishads.

Want to Know More About the Upanishads and Vedanta?

The Principal Upanishads. Translation by S. Radhakrishnan. New Delhi: Indus, 1995.

The Thirteen Principal Upanishads. Translation by Robert Hume. New York: Oxford University Press, 1979.

Upanishads. Translation by Patrick Olivelle. New York: Oxford University Press, 1996.

The Upanishads. Translation by Valerie Roebuck. New York: Penguin Books, 2000.

CHAPTER 4

Want to Know More About the Yoga Sutra?

OLD STANDBYS

Prabhavanda, Swami, and Christopher Isherwood. *How to Know God.* Hollywood, CA: Vedanta Press, 1953. *Supporting material: none.*

Taimni, I. K. *The Science of Yoga.* Wheaton, IL: Theosophical Publishing House, 1961. *Supporting material: nagari sutras and their Roman transliterations.*

INDIAN SCHOLARS/TEACHERS

Desikachar, T. K. V. *Reflections on the Yoga Sutras of Patanjali.* Chennai, India: Krishnamacharya Yoga Mandiram, 1987. *Supporting material: nagari sutras and their Roman transliterations; includes a CD with an audio rendition of the text chanted by Kausthub Desikachar.*

Hariharananda Aranya, Swami. *Yoga Philosophy of Patanjali.* Albany, NY: State University of New York, 1981. *Supporting material: appendices on jnana yoga, the tattvas, karma, glossary.*

Iyengar, B. K. S. *Light on the Yoga Sutras of Patanjali.* London: Aquarian/Thorsons, 1993. *Supporting material: nagari sutras and their Roman transliterations; thematic key to text, interconnection of the sutras, alphabetical index of sutras, yoga in a nutshell, glossary.*

WESTERN SCHOLARS/TEACHERS

Bouanchaud, Bernard. *The Essence of Yoga.* Portland, OR: Rudra Press, 1997. *Supporting material: themes for "personal reflection" for each sutra, glossary.*

Bryant, Edwin. *The Yoga Sutras of Patanjali*. New York: North Point Press, 2009. *Supporting material: nagari sutras and their Roman transliterations, chapter summaries, extensive notes.*

Chapple, Christopher, and Yogi Ananda Viraj. *The Yoga Sutras of Patanjali.* New Delhi: Sri Satguru Publications, 1990. *Supporting material: word-for-word breakdown, index of Sanskrit terms.*

Feuerstein, Georg. *The Yoga-Sutra of Patanjali*. Rochester, VT: Inner Traditions, 1989. *Supporting material: nagari sutras and their Roman transliterations, along with word-for-word breakdown; word index.*

Hartranft, Chip. *The Yoga-Sutra of Patanjali*. Boston: Shambhala, 2003. *Supporting material: a discussion of the text and its translation, an outline of the "Yogic Path," glossary, bibliography.*

Savitripriya, Swami. *Psychology of Mystical Awakening.* Sunnyvale, CA: New Life Books, 1991. *Supporting material: glossary.*

Stoler Miller, Barbara. *Yoga: Discipline of Freedom.* Berkeley, CA: University of California Press, 1995. *Supporting material: keywords in the text and in Sanskrit.*

SECONDARY SOURCES

Bachman, Nicolai. *The Path of the Yoga Sutras.* Boulder, CO: Sounds True, 2011.

Eliade, Mircea. *Patanjali and Yoga.* New York: Schocken Books, 1976.

Iyengar, B. K. S. *Core of the Yoga Sutras.* London: HarperThorsons, 2012.

White, David Gordon. *The Yoga Sutra of Patanjali: A Biography.* Princeton, NJ: Princeton University Press, 2014.

Want to Know More About Kundalini?

Avalon, Arthur [John Woodroffe]. *The Serpent Power*. New York: Dover, 1974.

Want to Know More About Placing?

Feuerstein, Georg. "Nyasa." In *The Encyclopedia of Yoga and Tantra,* 250–51. Boston: Shambhala, 2011.

Flood, Gavin. "The Divinisation of the Body." In *The Tantric Body,* 113–16. New York: I. B. Tauris, 2006.

CHAPTER 5

Want to Know More About Asana?

Buhnemann, Gudren. *Eighty-four Asanas in Yoga: A Survey of Traditions.* New Delhi, India: DK Printworld (P), Ltd., 2007.

Sjoman, N. E. *The Yoga Tradition of the Mysore Palace.* New Delhi, India: Abhinav Publications, 1996.

Want to Know More About Sun Salutation?

Balasahib Pandit Pratinidhi, Shrimant. *The Ten-Point Way to Health.* London: J. M. Dent, 1938.

Jois, K. Pattabhi. "Surya Namaskara." In *Yoga Mala,* 34–47. New York: Northpoint Press, 1999.

Satyananda Sarasvati, Swami. *Surya Namaskara: A Technique of Solar Vitalization.* Munger, Bihar, India: Bihar School of Yoga, 1996.

Want to Know More About Props?

Shifroni, Eyal. *A Chair for Yoga: A Complete Guide to Iyengar Yoga Practice with a Chair.* Privately printed, 2013. www.eyalshifroni.com/shop

———. *Props for Yoga.* Vol. 1, *Standing Asanas.* Privately printed, 2015. www.eyalshifroni.com/shop

Want to Know More About Mantra?

Alper, Harvey, ed. *Mantra.* Albany, NY: State University of New York, 1989.

Beck, Guy. *Sonic Theology: Hinduism and Sacred Sound.* Columbia, SC: University of South Carolina Press, 1993.

Padoux, Andre. *Vac: The Concept of the Word in Selected Hindu Tantras.* Albany, NY: State University of New York, 1990.

Want to Know More About Hatha Meditation?

Along with the *Shiva Samhita,* the other two of the Big Three traditional Hatha Yoga books, the *Hatha Yoga Pradipika* and the *Gheranda Samhita,* both describe meditation practices. See chapter 4 of the *Hatha Yoga Pradipika,* and chapters 6 and 7 of the *Gheranda Samhita.* If you're interested in this subject, you might also seek out an online copy of the Yoga Upanishads (see Chapter 4), in which you'll find many engaging ideas for meditation.

Want to Know More About the Literature of Hatha Yoga?

900–1000 C.E.

Discussion of Knowledge Pertaining to the Kaula Tradition (Kaula Jnana Nirnaya). Varanasi, India: Prachya Prakashan, 2007.

1000–1100 C.E.

Gharote, M. L., and G. K. Pai, eds. *Doctrine of the Adepts' Tracks* (*Siddha Siddhanta Paddhati*). Lonavla, India: Lonavla Yoga Institute, 2010.

1200–1300 C.E.

Feuerstein, Georg. *Goraksha's Tracks* (*Goraksha Paddhati*). In *The Yoga Tradition*, 532–59. Prescott, AZ: Hohm Press, 1998.
Yajnavalkya's Yoga (*Yoga Yajnavalkya*), translated by A. G. Mohan. Madras: Ganesh & Co., n.d.

1300–1400 C.E.

Amanaska Yoga, translated by Jason Birch, November 2006. http://nathi.ru /read/books/TheAmanaskaYogaVersion4.pdf
Seed of Yoga (*Yoga Bija*). Delhi, India: Swami Keshwananda Yoga Institute, n.d.
Trans-minded Yoga (*Amanaska Yoga*). Delhi: Swami Keshawananda Yoga Samsthan Prakashana, 1987.

1400–1500 C.E.

Light on Hatha Yoga (*Hatha Yoga Pradipika*). www.YogaVidya.com. (2002)
Sparkling Lines on Yoga (*Yoga Taravali*). Chennai, India: Krishnamacharya Yoga Mandiram. (2003)

1500–1600 C.E.

Song of the "Shaken Off" (*Avadhuta Gita*). Madras, India: Sri Ramakrishna Math, n.d.

1600–1700 C.E.

Gheranda's Compendium (*Gheranda Samhita*). www.Yoga.Vidya.com. (2004)
Shiva's Compendium (*Shiva Samhita*). www.Yoga.Vidya.com. (2007)
String of Jewels on Hatha [Yoga] (*Hatha Ratna Avali*). Lonavla, India: Lonavla Yoga Institute, n.d.

1700–1800 C.E.

Great Blowout Tantra (*Mahanirvana Tantra*). New York: Dover, 1972.
Investigation of the Six Centers (*Shat Cakra Nirupani*). In *The Serpent Power,* by Arthur Avalon [John Woodroffe]. New York: Dover, 1974.
Moonlight on the Principles of Hatha [Yoga] (*Hatha Tattva Kaumudi*). Lonavla, India: Lonavla Yoga Institute, n.d.

All twenty-one of the Yoga Upanishads are available for free at (though the translation is uneven): http://archive.org/details/TheYogaUpanishads. You can find three of these texts (*Amrita Nada Bindu, Advaya Taraka,* and *Kshurika*) in Chapter 15 of Georg Feuerstein's *The Yoga Tradition.* Also in this classic volume is a selection from the *Flood of Kula Tantra (Kularnava Tantra)* and the entire text of *Goraksha's Tracks (Goraksha Paddhati).*

Secondary sources

Burley, Mikel. *Hatha-Yoga.* New Delhi: Motilal Banaridass, 2000.

de Michelis, Elizabeth. *A History of Modern Yoga.* London: Continuum, 2005.

Singleton, Mark. *Yoga Body.* Oxford: Oxford University Press, 2010.

Sivananda Radha, Swami. *Hatha Yoga: The Hidden Language.* Porthill, ID: Timeless Books, 1987.

White, David Gordon. *The Alchemical Body.* Chicago: University of Chicago Press, 1996.

Index

Hatha Yoga and, 10, 145, 196–97
mudras and, 201
overview, 148–50
Patanjali and, 93
prana and, 169, 196
pranayama and, 196–98
root cakra and, 145, 196, 203
and samadhi, 145, 200
Shakti and, 148–49, 196
Veda Bharati on, 93

language, xvi–xvii, 71. *See also* Sanskrit
Larson, Gerald, 13, 114
left hand, 160
Lewis, James, 21–22
Light on Yoga (Iyengar), 61, 192, 213
peacock misprint in, 59–60
Lorenzen, David, 115–16

madhyama shabda, 207
maha mudra, 71
maha siddhi, 113–14
Maitra, Lakshmi Kanta, 48
Maitreyi, 78–79
Maitri Upanishad, 37–38, 137, 138, 208
mantras, 156, 158–61, 188–89, 211
cakras and, 147, 159
nature of, 209–10
Patanjali on, 121
in *Rig Veda*, 25, 81, 123, 184
in sandhya rite, 151
unspoken mantra, 210–11
in *Yajur Veda*, 184, 185
Yoga Sutra and, 113
See also OM
Marshall, John, 23, 24
Masson, Charles. See Lewis, James
mats, 154–55
Maurer, Walter, 49, 54–58
maya, 83–84
meditation, 17, 122, 147, 152, 213–14
Meru, 141–43
Meru Danda, 141, 181
midnight practice, 153
Mittra, Dharma, 61
Mohenjo Daro, 22–24
moksha, 153, 173
monism, 11, 83
vs. dualism, 12, 28
morning practice, 151–53

mudras, 146, 152
asanas and, 223
bandhas and, 180, 196, 200
categories of, 200–201
hasta, 71, 184
Hatha Yoga and, 223
namaste and, 221
nature of, 200
pranayama and, 196, 200–201, 223
Shoulder Stand as mudra, 173–74
muladhara cakra, 147
Müller, Max, 43, 49
Mundaka Upanishad, 76

nada, 152–53
Nada Yoga, 152, 208–9
nadi shodhana, 131
nadis, 144–45, 158, 208
asana(s) and, 144, 145, 173, 208
Hatha Yoga and, 78, 133, 143–44
nature of, 143–45
prana and, 78, 133, 143–45, 169
See also ida nadi; pingala nadi; sushumna
nadi
nagari, 147, 158, 159
devanagari and, 49
interpretations of, 49
punctuation in, 62
pundit/pandit and, 52
Sanskrit and, 49–51, 55, 56, 58, 59, 182
sibilants, 55
spelling and roots of the word, 55, 56
namaste, 220–21
nirodha, 26, 195–96
niyamas, 20, 103–6, 168, 218–20
nothing, thinking of, 214–15
numbers, sacred, 170–72
nyasa, 158–61

observances. *See* niyamas
Olivelle, Patrick, 74, 76
OM, 19, 20, 76, 78, 210–12. *See also* pranava
oshadhi, 122–23
Ouspensky, Peter, 128

Panini, 47–48
Parable of the Chariot (*Ratha Kalpana*),
8–10
partridge and the horse (story), 77–78

subtle anatomy of yoga, 138–41
Sun-Moon, 131–33. *See also* hatha
Sun Salutation, age of, 183–87
sushumna nadi, 133, 143, 144–47, 150, 178,
    180, 196, 203, 209
sutkas, 65–68
sutra atman, 25
sutra(s), 85–86, 95, 97
    as aphorism, 86–88
    nature of, 86, 87, 97
svadhyaya, 20, 104, 108–9
Svatmarama, 80, 164, 170–73, 179, 214, 218,
    221
    on breathing, 131, 133, 199
    on Hatha Yoga, 135, 164
    on matha, 164
    Nada Yoga and, 208–9
    Patanjali and, 135
    on practice and poses, 16–17, 131–33, 148,
        152, 173, 175, 208, 218
    pranayama and, 133, 148, 152, 173, 198
    on Raja Yoga, 135
    See also Hatha Yoga Pradipika
swami/svami, 2

Taittiriya Upanishad, 12
tapas, 104, 113, 164
    nature of, 109–10
thinking of nothing, 214–15
Tiger Pose, 61
time, linear vs. cyclical, 66
*Tri Shikhi Brahmana Upanishad (Triple Tuft
    Brahmana Upanishad)*, 168
Tyberg, Judith, 67

union, 10–11
    yoga and, 6–7, 12–14
union-method, yoga as, 7–8
"upanishad," meaning of the word, 72–75
upanishadic categories, 78
Upanishads, 4, 75–76, 78, 167–68
    Arthur Schopenhauer on, 4
    authors of, 79–80
    Brahma Vidya Upanishad, 37, 81
    Brahman and, 11, 167
    Brahmanas and, 83, 168
    nadis and, 144
    number of, 75–77
    overview and nature of, 63, 71–72
    Vedanta and, 82, 83

Vedas and, 63, 71, 72, 75, 76, 83, 109
    women in, 78–79
utkata, 178–79
uttanasana, 180

vac, 206–8
vairagya, 125
vayus, 202, 203
Veda Bharati, Swami, 2, 25, 93
Vedanta, 28, 71, 73, 101
    Hatha Yoga and, 222
    meaning of the word, 83
    nature of, 82–84
Vedanta Sutra, 82, 109, 172
Vedas, 11, 43, 83, 108
    age, 65–66
    Garuda and, 182
    Hatha Yoga compared with, 218, 219
    overview and nature of, 63–67
    root and meaning of the word, 63
    Sri Aurobindo on, 67
    Sun Salutation and, 185
    sutkas in, 212
    Upanishads and, 63, 71–72, 75–76, 83,
        109
    Vyasa and, 95
    See also Rig Veda; Yajur Veda
"Viagra" as derived from the word *vyaghra*
    (tiger), 60–61
vibhuti, 112–13
viparita karani mudra, 152, 174–76, 218
visarga, 57, 160
Vishnu, 29–30, 176–77
viveka, 124–26
Vivekananda, Swami, 36, 134–35
viyoga, 13
vṛtti, 8, 100, 195, 201, 204, 211
vyaghra, "Viagra" as derived from the word,
    60–61
Vyasa, 9, 94–97, 113
    Yoga Sutra and, 9, 164–65, 207, 217

Walker, Benjamin, 49
Westerners, yoga's appropriateness for, xv,
    3–6
White, David Gordon, 23–24, 97
Whitney, William, 42–43, 56
wind, Sanskrit words for, 203
Winternitz, Maurice, 47, 69–71, 76
Woodroffe, John, 143, 159, 183

About the Author

RICHARD ROSEN began his practice of Hatha Yoga in 1980 at the Yoga Room in Berkeley, California, and from 1982 to 1985 he trained at the BKS Iyengar Yoga Institute in San Francisco. In 1987 he cofounded the Piedmont Yoga Studio with his good friends Clare Finn and Rodney Yee, and taught there for nearly twenty-eight years until it closed its doors in January 2015. He continues to teach at the same location, now called You and the Mat. Richard is a contributing editor at *Yoga Journal* magazine, and since 1990 he's written feature articles, book reviews, a variety of columns, and more than three hundred yoga video reviews. He's also the author of four books, *The Yoga of Breath* (Shambhala 2002), *Yoga for 50+* (Ulysses 2004), *Pranayama beyond the Fundamentals* (Shambhala 2006), and *Original Yoga* (Shambhala 2012), and has recorded a seven-CD set titled *The Practice of Pranayama* (Shambhala 2010). Since 1989 he's been on the board of directors of the California Yoga Teachers Association, and in 2008 helped form CYTA's grant-making wing, the Yoga Dana Foundation, which supports California yoga teachers working with underserved populations, such as at-risk and incarcerated youth and disabled students. Richard lives in a cottage built in 1906 in beautiful Berkeley.